Vascular Access in Neonatal Nursing
Practice: A Neuroprotective Approach

Matheus Roland van Rens • Kevin Hugill

Vascular Access in Neonatal Nursing Practice: A Neuroprotective Approach

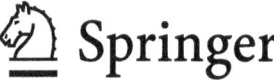 Springer

Matheus Roland van Rens
Neonatal Intensive Care Unit
Radboud University Medical Center,
Amalia Children's Hospital
Nijmegen, The Netherlands

Kevin Hugill
Formerly Director of Nursing Education
Hamad Medical Corporation
Doha, Qatar

ISBN 978-3-031-81601-7   ISBN 978-3-031-81602-4   (eBook)
https://doi.org/10.1007/978-3-031-81602-4

This Springer imprint is published by the registered company Springer Nature Switzerland AG
The registered company address is: Gewerbestrasse 11, 6330 Cham, Switzerland

If disposing of this product, please recycle the paper.

Preface

The gestation of this book has been prolonged and has evolved out of discussions over several years between the authors. These explorations highlighted unrealised opportunities to better integrate vascular access into overall care and the considerable variations seen in everyday vascular access practice. These variations in practice were often based on established habits unsupported by research evidence; a situation that was both frustrating and affecting the quality of care.

Since the onset of neonatal care as a discrete subspecialty of health care, vascular access has established a fundamental role in providing therapies. In more recent decades, the benefits of using developmentally supportive concepts and frameworks and integrating families into care have become firmly established. However, despite its centrality, practices around obtaining and using vascular access have not always been given the attention they deserve within neonatal care and are often viewed in isolation, leading to fragmented care. This book sets out to establish vascular access practice within a wider neuroprotective and developmental supportive stance. This book is for everyone who wants to promote better integrated and less fragmented care for infants and their families.

The authors have many decades of experience in neonatology and hold advanced academic and practice qualifications. They have held academic, clinical, and managerial positions across Europe and the Middle East and have personal experience of preterm birth. These experiences which have informed their practice and thinking. Together and separately, they have presented at international conferences and workshops and have published widely on neonatal topics. In addition, both are active members of the Neonatal European Vascular Access Team (NEVAT), a key Europe wide inter-professional organisation for the advancement of better neonatal vascular access.

This book is directed at a wide audience of neonatal nurses and other healthcare professionals involved in providing and using vascular access for preterm and sick newborn infants. Individual chapters address key topics and summarise essential elements of the evidence supporting practice and identify gaps in knowledge. To encourage readers to reflect upon and assimilate this information, practice point text boxes and directed case studies based on real-world events are included in each chapter.

By bringing together vascular access, neuroprotective, developmental, and family involvement considerations, the authors hope to stimulate readers to reflect and consider changes in their own and their organisation's thinking and practices. Our shared view is that doing this can make vascular access more visible, leading to better integration with wider care considerations and care delivery, which could lead to potentially better outcomes.

Almansa, Spain   Matheus Roland van Rens
Cumbria, UK   Kevin Hugill

Contents

1   **Introduction to the Book**   1
     1.1   Rationale for the Book   1
     1.2   Why Is Vascular Access Important?   2
     1.3   Layout of This Book   3
     References   4

**Part I   General Considerations for Neonatal Vascular
             Access Within a Neuroprotective Stance**

2   **Neonatal Vascular Access: An Overview
     of Its Unique Aspects**   7
     2.1   Introduction   7
     2.2   Historical Perspectives on the Development
          of Vascular Access   8
     2.3   Defining the Uniqueness of Neonatal Vascular Access   9
          2.3.1   Neonatal Anatomy   10
          2.3.2   Neonatal Physiology   11
     2.4   Approaches to Infection Prevention
          During Vascular Access   14
     2.5   Integrating Neuroprotective Measures and Integrating
          Families in Vascular Access   15
          2.5.1   Parents' Experiences   15
          2.5.2   Developmentally Sensitive Care Practices   15
     2.6   Planning for Vascular Access Needs   18
          2.6.1   Constructing an n-VAMP   19
          2.6.2   Factors to Consider When Deciding
                 on Which Intravenous Access Device   22
     2.7   Terminologies Used in This Book   24
          2.7.1   Vascular Access Devices   24
     2.8   Concluding Remarks   25
     References   26

Part II   Optimising Neonatal Vascular Access

3   Technology in Vascular Access   35
   3.1   Introduction   35
       3.1.1   Impacts of Technology   36
   3.2   Technological Approaches to Vascular Access Device
       Design and Manufacture   37
       3.2.1   Catheter Design and Material   37
       3.2.2   Advanced Design Features   39
   3.3   Technological Approaches for Ensuring Safe Insertion
       of Vascular Access Devices   42
       3.3.1   Aiding Better PVAD Insertion   42
       3.3.2   Aiding Better CVAD Insertion   44
       3.3.3   Aiding Better Securement of PVADs and CVADs   46
   3.4   Technological Aids Ensuring Safe Infusion   48
       3.4.1   Sensing Technologies   48
   3.5   Technology and Its Impacts on NICU Parents   49
   3.6   Concluding Remarks   51
   References   52

Part III   Insertion, Use, and Aftercare of Vascular Access Devices

4   Peripheral Vascular Access Device Insertion   61
   4.1   Introduction   61
   4.2   Selecting the Appropriate Vessel for PVAD Placement   62
       4.2.1   Vein Assessment   62
       4.2.2   Difficult Intravenous Access (DIVA)   62
   4.3   Ensuring Safe PVAD Insertion   63
       4.3.1   Skin Preparation   63
       4.3.2   Insertion Techniques   65
       4.3.3   Preventing Pain and Promoting Comfort
           during PVAD Insertion   66
   4.4   Sealing, Securement, Stabilisation, and Exit Site Dressing   70
       4.4.1   Cyanoacrylate Tissue Adhesive   71
       4.4.2   Splints   72
   4.5   Concluding Remarks   74
   References   77

5   Peripheral Vascular Access Care and Management   83
   5.1   Introduction   83
       5.1.1   Overview   84
   5.2   Supporting Safe Infusion Therapy   84
       5.2.1   Smart Infusion Systems   86
       5.2.2   Alarm Fatigue   88
       5.2.3   In-Line Pressure Monitoring   88
       5.2.4   Managing Occlusion Pump Alarms   89

5.3   PVAD Complications.   91
       5.3.1   Leaks and Accidental Removals   92
5.4   Infusion Site Monitoring for the Early Detection
       of Complications   92
       5.4.1   Touch–Look–Compare (TLC)   92
       5.4.2   ivWatch   94
5.5   Phlebitis   94
5.6   Medical Adhesive Related Skin Injury (MARSI)   94
5.7   Peripheral Intravenous Infiltration Extravasation (PIVIE).   95
       5.7.1   Signs of PIVIE.   96
       5.7.2   Determining the Severity of PIVIE   96
       5.7.3   Treating PIVIE.   97
5.8   Concluding Remarks   100
References.   102

6   **Central Vascular Access Devices**   107
6.1   Introduction   107
6.2   Selecting the Most Appropriate CVAD   109
       6.2.1   N-PICC/ECC   110
       6.2.2   CICC and FICC   110
6.3   Selecting the Appropriate Vessel for CVAD Placement.   110
       6.3.1   Blood Vessel Suitability Assessment   111
       6.3.2   Catheter-to-Vein Ratio   112
       6.3.3   Catheter Sizing.   113
6.4   CVAD Insertion   113
       6.4.1   Reducing Infection Risk During CVAD Insertion   114
       6.4.2   CVAD Insertion Techniques   115
       6.4.3   MST in n-PICC/ECC.   116
6.5   Securement and Dressing.   118
6.6   Complications   119
       6.6.1   CLABSI   122
6.7   Promoting Comfort, Relieving Pain, and Involving Parents   124
       6.7.1   Parent Involvement   125
6.8   Concluding Remarks   126
References.   128

7   **Specialist Vascular Access Devices**.   137
7.1   Introduction   137
7.2   Umbilical Vascular Catheters.   138
       7.2.1   Umbilical Vein Catheters (UVC).   138
       7.2.2   Umbilical Arterial Catheters (UAC)   139
7.3   Intra-Arterial Catheters (IAC)   144
       7.3.1   Upper Limb IAC   144
       7.3.2   Lower Limb IAC   144
       7.3.3   IAC Insertion, Securement, and Removal   147
       7.3.4   Complications Associated with IAC   147

7.4   Intraosseous (IO) Access to the Circulation.   149
       7.4.1   Complications Associated with IO Devices.   149
7.5   Vascular Access in Specialist Situations   151
       7.5.1   Advanced Extracorporeal Life Support   151
7.6   Concluding Remarks   153
References.   155

Part IV   Neonatal Vascular Access in Context

**8   Integrating Neonatal Vascular Access
       and Neuroprotective Care**   163
8.1   Introduction   163
8.2   The Origins of Parental Centeredness
       and Family Integration.   164
       8.2.1   Parents' Concerns   165
8.3   Doing Things to Help Integrate Vascular
       and Neuroprotective Care   166
       8.3.1   Parents' Needs in Vascular Access.   166
       8.3.2   Infants' Needs in Vascular Access   169
       8.3.3   Organisational Needs in Vascular Access   171
       8.3.4   Looking to the Future.   172
8.4   Final Thoughts   174
       8.4.1   Questions for Research   174
       8.4.2   Bringing It all Together and Defragmenting Care   176
References.   179

Introduction to the Book

1

This book provides a unique resource for nurses and other healthcare providers at all levels involved in obtaining, using, and managing neonatal vascular access. *Vascular Access in Neonatal Nursing Practice, A Neuroprotective Approach* provides a combination of theory, research evidence, and practice insights integrated with the essential principles of neuroprotective and family-integrated care.

1.1 Rationale for the Book

This book considers the topic of vascular access in neonates, an issue of considerable relevance to nurses and other healthcare providers working in neonatal care settings. Despite this, neonatal vascular access is an aspect of practice whose evidence-base is with some exceptions underdeveloped, lacking in standardisation, and whose integration into overall care delivery and planning is largely ignored. The inspiration for this book arose out of our extensive contacts over many years with infants and their families across the world having vascular access procedures, including care delivery, service management, education, and research. These experiences have convinced us that there is a desire amongst many nurses and parents that we can and should do things better than we currently do. Consequently, to achieve this ambition, neonatal vascular access deserves a higher profile; this book is a part of this endeavour.

The uniqueness of neonatal anatomy and physiology, and health professionals choices and behaviours directly affect the success of vascular access. The utility of neuroprotective measures has become increasingly legitimate in many aspects of neonatal care, and whilst vascular access research has provided much needed evidence about better practices, the two are often viewed as independent areas of study. We believe that integrating neuroprotective interventions and concepts of family integrative care into how we carry out vascular access procedures can make a

© The Author(s), under exclusive license to Springer Nature Switzerland AG 2024
M. R. van Rens, K. Hugill, *Vascular Access in Neonatal Nursing Practice:
A Neuroprotective Approach*, https://doi.org/10.1007/978-3-031-81602-4_1

significant contribution to improving vascular access practices. This view about how care can be organised and delivered has the potential to positively affect patient and family outcomes in diverse and far-reaching ways. In effect, the outcomes and experiences of vascular access for infants and their families would be better if they were coordinated with and integrated with wider neuroprotective approaches. In this book, we aim to link the theory, research, and practice of vascular access within a larger neuroprotective paradigm of care in an informative and authoritative, yet accessible and relevant way.

1.2   Why Is Vascular Access Important?

Repeated vascular access procedures to access the circulation for the administration of therapies or diagnostic blood sampling are a pervasive, uncomfortable, and often painful experience for most preterm and sick infants admitted to neonatal intensive care units (NICUs) across the world [1–3]. Some estimates suggest that infants in NICU experience on average painful procedures numbering around the mid-teens daily [3, 4]. However, the accuracy of such figures should be treated with caution as they vary considerably. The figures depend upon definitional differences about what constitutes a painful procedure and how they are counted (e.g., direct observation versus self-reports). Estimates of the overall number of skin breaking procedures associated with vascular access also vary. To some extent, these figures are influenced by first-attempt insertion success rates and the frequency of complications. It is likely that both insertion success rates and complications are underreported due to varying documentation practices, lack of standardised reporting protocols, and the inherent challenges in tracking all adverse events.

Regardless of the actual number, the adverse effects of repeated painful experiences are thought to be accumulative and associated with adverse short- and long-term developmental outcomes [5–7]. Interventions that promote comfort and reduce overall pain experience are to be welcomed. In addition, care models and frameworks that lead to better integration of vascular access into overall care whilst facilitating greater incorporation of families into care should be promoted. Despite the essential and often critical importance of vascular access amongst neonates, it is associated with a high burden of risk and complications (e.g., [1, 2, 8, 9]) and often perceived as a reactive response to pressing needs rather than as part of proactive, pre-planned, and integrated facet of overall care. To achieve better outcomes and experiences for infants and their families, this situation is untenable and the importance of ensuring better vascular access needs to be acknowledged more widely.

1.3   Layout of This Book

The book is organised around three sections: 'General Considerations for Neonatal Vascular Access', 'Optimising Neonatal Vascular Access', and 'Insertion, Use, and Aftercare of Vascular Access Devices', which reflect the focus of the individual chapters within them. Each of the chapters, after this introductory chapter which sets out key aspects of the book's structure (e.g., Text Box 1.1) explores a particular focus on neonatal vascular access and incorporates text boxes that summarise important practice points. Towards the end of each chapter are the summary key points, and topic-relevant case histories based on real-life events together with reflective questions and exercises which are intended to encourage readers to reflect upon their own practice and to embed the material in this book into their everyday practice.

Chapter 2 provides an overview of the unique aspects of practice affecting neonatal vascular access and of the developmental challenges faced in neonatal care and how practitioners have responded to these. Key concepts of neuroprotective and family-integrated care area are delineated, and consideration is given as to how these perspectives can be better utilised within vascular access. In doing this, this chapter develops the overarching context for much of the subsequent discussion. Also, in this chapter, neonatal vascular access management planning (n-VAMP) is considered. This is a significant innovation that has the potential to influence the way that vascular access practice can evolve to better meet the needs of infants and their families. Chapter 3 explores the contributions and application of technology in supporting vascular access, including technology to aid the optimum choice of blood vessel, device, insertion technique, device fixation, and aftercare.

Chapters 4, 5, and 6 consider the insertion, use, and aftercare of the various vascular catheters commonly used in neonatal practice, applying proven neuroprotective strategies aimed at improving the experience of infants and parents. Chapter 4 focuses on issues around peripheral vascular device insertion, a significant area of vascular access where nurses often take the lead. Chapter 5 continues the peripheral vascular access focus and considers safe infusion therapy and the prevention, detection, and management of complications associated with peripheral devices.

In Chap. 6, the topic of focus moves to central vascular access devices with a particular emphasis on neonatal-peripherally inserted central catheters, also referred to as epicutaneo-caval catheters (n-PICC/ECC) insertion. Chapter 7 explores some of the alternate choices for vascular access in neonates combining consideration of umbilical catheters, intra-arterial catheters, and intraosseous devices. Finally, Chap. 8 reviews the key themes highlighted within this book. We look to the future both in relation to practice and the opportunities from increased integration of vascular access practice within a neuroprotective, developmental, and family-integrated stance. We draw together the research and educational literature and make it relevant to practice. The reflective exercise in this chapter asks the reader to consider the effects of their own vascular access practice and how it affects infants and families in their care and consider how best to balance the drivers for best vascular access practice and their interactions with families.

Text Box 1.1 Inclusive Language
In writing this book, we acknowledge the effect language can have on individuals and populations. We recognise that individual identity is socially constructed, and expression varies from person to person. Whilst there may be cultural expectations, everyone will have their own internal view of what their identity means and feels like for them.

In this book, we use the term 'nurse' and 'healthcare provider' (doctor, surgeon, pharmacist, psychologist, dietician, etc.) to imply persons who have undergone a prescribed period of education, preparation, and assessment to be recognised as holding these professional roles within their regulatory authority's jurisdiction. Unless explicitly stated otherwise, when reporting on research studies, we use the word 'parent' to imply 'mothers', 'fathers',' primary carers', and 'legal guardians' inclusively as people providing care to another regardless of biological relationships, disability, age, health status, race, ethnicity, sexual orientation, gender, religion, or politics.

References

1. Legemaat M, Carr PJ, van Rens MFPT, Van Dijk M, Poslawsky IE, van den Hoogen A. Peripheral intravenous cannulation: complication rates in the neonatal population: a multicenter observational study. J Vasc Access. 2016;17(4):360–5. https://doi.org/10.5301/jva.5000558.
2. van Rens MFPT, Hugill K, Mahmah MA, Bayoumi M, Francia ALV, Garcia KLP, et al. Evaluation of unmodifiable and potentially modifiable factors affecting peripheral intravenous device-related complications in neonates: a retrospective observational study. BMJ Open. 2021;11(9):e047788. https://doi.org/10.1136/bmjopen-2020-047788.
3. Carbajal R, Rousset A, Danan C, Coquery S, Nolent P, Ducrocq S, et al. Epidemiology and treatment of painful procedures in neonates in intensive care units. JAMA. 2008;300(1):60–70. https://doi.org/10.1001/jama.300.1.60.
4. Simons SH, van Dijk M, Anand KS, Roofthooft D, van Lingen RA, Tibboel D. Do we still hurt newborn babies? A prospective study of procedural pain and analgesia in neonates. Arch Pediatr Adolesc Med. 2003;157(11):1058–64. https://doi.org/10.1001/archpedi.157.11.1058.
5. Valeri BO, Holsti L, Linhares MB. Neonatal pain and developmental outcomes in children born preterm. Clin J Pain. 2015;3(4):355–62. https://doi.org/10.1097/AJP.0000000000000114.
6. Pereira FL, Gaspardo CM. Neonatal pain and developmental outcomes in children born preterm. Psychol Neurosci. 2024;17(1):1–15. https://doi.org/10.1037/pne0000332.
7. Weber A, Harrison TM. Reducing toxic stress in the NICU to improve infant outcomes. Nurs Outlook. 2019;67(2):169–89. https://doi.org/10.1016/j.outlook.2018.11.002.
8. Arnts IJJ, Bullens LM, Groenewoud JMM, Liem KD. Comparison of complication rates between umbilical and peripherally inserted central venous catheters in newborns. J Obstet Gynecol Neonat Nurs. 2014;43(2):205–15. https://doi.org/10.1111/1552-6909.12278.
9. Pet GC, Eickhoff JC, McNevin KE, Do J, McAdams RM. Risk factors for peripherally inserted central catheter complications in neonates. J Perinatol. 2020;40(4):581–8. https://doi.org/10.1038/s41372-019-0575-7.

Part I

General Considerations for Neonatal Vascular Access Within a Neuroprotective Stance

Neonatal Vascular Access: An Overview of Its Unique Aspects

2

Chapter Learning Objectives
Upon completing this chapter, readers will be able to:

- Critically appraise the impacts of neonatal anatomy and physiology on vascular access.
- Implement the foundational principles of infection control and aseptic technique into neonatal vascular access procedures.
- Evaluate the emotional and psychological impacts on parents of neonatal vascular access procedures.
- Advocate for the use of neuroprotective measures and family involvement during neonatal vascular access.
- Critically reflect on the potential benefits to clinical practice and infant experience from developing individualised neonatal vascular access management plans (n-VAMP).
- Utilise a standardised typology of vascular access devices.

2.1   Introduction

Vascular access is a critical aspect of caring for newborn infants in various clinical settings, including neonatal intensive care units (NICUs), delivery rooms, and emergency departments. However, proving safe and effective vascular access for this patient population presents unique challenges and complexities. Some of which relate to their anatomy and physiology, the impacts of preterm birth, infant's developmental stage, and how healthcare provider decisions and behaviours can inadvertently have undesired psychological and developmental consequences. This situation differentiates infants in neonatal intensive care units (NICUs) from older patient groups and necessitates the need to adapt existing practices or apply specialised approaches and techniques. Understanding these considerations is crucial for nurses

© The Author(s), under exclusive license to Springer Nature Switzerland AG 2024
M. R. van Rens, K. Hugill, *Vascular Access in Neonatal Nursing Practice: A Neuroprotective Approach*, https://doi.org/10.1007/978-3-031-81602-4_2

to enable them to adapt and apply the tenets of pervading ideas about developmentally protective and parent/family supporting care to deliver optimal vascular access care and minimise complications.

2.2   Historical Perspectives on the Development of Vascular Access

Reports of experimentation in vascular access have a very long history dating back to antiquity, with many claims and counter claims of discovery, invention, and 'firsts' [1, 2]. Somewhat concerningly, some of these early milestones predated modern medical knowledge of anatomy, physiology, pharmacology, bacteriology, and infection prevention. Clinical use of intravenous therapy was often limited by a lack of suitable equipment [3, 4]. The late nineteenth and early twentieth century saw the invention and proliferation of various designs of vascular access devices and catheters. However, some of these were associated with serious complications and were of limited utility and consequently rejected by an unready medical establishment [4]. The introduction of glass syringes, high-quality hollow steel needles drove the increased acceptance of infusion-based therapies as a therapeutic option [4, 5], even in some neonatal settings [6–8]. However, several factors precluded universal use away from leading centres of healthcare, including:

- Small-scale specialist manufacture of often incompatible designs.
- Needle migration and breakage puncturing blood vessel walls.
- Risks of inadvertent arterial puncture.
- Limited availability of safe parenteral drug formulations free from hazardous excipients.

From the late 1950s and early 1960s onwards, reliable single use plastic equipment, which was sterilised at the point of manufacture became widely available [4, 5]. This progress, particularly in the hospitals of high-income nations coupled with industrial-scale pharmaceutical developments, was instrumental in increasing the reliability and safety of infusion therapy. A development that resulted in the increased routinisation of vascular access (especially peripheral) and infusion-based therapies across all patient groups including the newborn. As one pioneer of neonatal care, Professor Harold Gamsu reflecting on earlier times noted in 1999:

> It should be said that the development of reliable and disposable equipment was one of the major reasons for improvement in neonatal care. Sharp and fine needles, plastic syringes with the plunger moving smoothly in the barrel predictably... [9, p. 35].

The significant improvements in survival outcomes for preterm infants in the 'pre-surfactant era' were also supported by new technology suitable for analysing micro blood samples. The results of these diagnostic tests enabled the targeted correction of metabolic imbalances using intravenous fluid therapy, themselves key factors in improvements in neonatal mortality and morbidity outcomes [9].

First-generation peripheral vascular catheters were comprised of a flexible synthetic plastic polymer (polyvinyl chloride, PVC) tube over a metal introducer stylet. These designs were based upon the work of Massa and collaborators [10]. Later generations incorporated new materials, including polytetrafluoroethylene (PTFE), marketed under the trade name Teflon™, fluorinated ethylene polypropylene (FEP), polyether block amide (PEBA), and polyurethane polymers (PUR). Further design improvements such as the addition of 'wings' to aid in inserter handling and device stabilisation and fixation, flashback visualisation windows to confirm lumen entry, shrouded needle safety devices to protect from needlestick injury have become commonplace. More recently, closed infusion systems, or antimicrobial coating/impregnation technology intended to prevent catheter-related bloodstream infection have become optional features for both peripheral and central vascular access devices and catheters [11].

The production of vascular access catheters optimised for use with the smallest neonatal patients has lagged those in other patient groups. This is partly due to unmet technical challenges and consequently steel hollow needles continued to be used in some neonatal care settings across the world until relatively recent times despite their limitations. More recent innovations compatible with the smaller diameter lumen of neonatal blood vessels have become increasingly used in practice. These devices, manufactured from chemical materials having thermoplastic properties reactive to body temperature, easing insertion and use, and reducing mechanical complications have proved to be particularly beneficial for NICU patients requiring peripheral vascular access [11–14]. Similar developments in the design and use of central venous access devices (CVAD), particularly neonatal-peripherally inserted central catheters (n-PICCs) also known as epicutaneo-cava catheters (ECCs), central and femorally inserted central catheter (CICC, FICC) have occurred in parallel [15, 16].

Traditionally, n-PICC/ECCs were inserted into superficial peripheral veins and threaded through the vasculature into a central vein using a combination of splitting needle or peelable cannula aids. More recently, micro-sized modified Seldinger technique (MST) insertion kits suitable for use in preterm blood vessel lumens have become available [17]. n-PICC/ECC catheter materials generally comprise polyurethane or silicone. However, silicone catheters have been largely abandoned in practice due to their greater fragility and risk of breakage, and poorer flow performance compared to polyurethane catheters [16]. Newer designs such as the incorporation of multiple lumens, closed infusion systems, antithrombotic and anti-infective technologies into catheters suitable for neonatal patients are commercially available, but evaluations of their benefits are mixed and further research is required to evidence their usefulness [18–20].

2.3 Defining the Uniqueness of Neonatal Vascular Access

Neonatal vascular access presents unique challenges, in part due to the innate attributes of newborn infants such as gestational age, weight, and particularities of their anatomy and physiology [21]. To provide safe and effective care to this vulnerable population, nurses and healthcare professionals must understand the distinctive features of newborn infant anatomical and physiological factors and their impacts on practice.

2.3.1 Neonatal Anatomy

Neonates have anatomical characteristics that pose challenges during vascular access procedures. The considerable variation in the weight and size of patients in NICUs further adds to this challenge. Infant weight at birth can range from a few hundred grams to over 4 kg, each circumstance presenting its own challenges for vascular access. Generally, peripheral blood vessels in those born preterm or with low birth weight are more mobile due to a relative lack of connective tissue and subcutaneous fat deposition, are physically smaller in size, having narrower lumens and thinner tissue layers, and are situated much closer to the skin surface (which is itself thinner and not fully matured). These features can limit vessel choice options, make it difficult to distinguish peripheral veins and arteries and identify suitable vessels for device placement and increase the likelihood of failed insertion or complications such as infiltration and extravasation [21–24].

Typically, infant blood volumes are slightly higher than older peoples' when calculated on a volume per kilogram weight basis, in the order of 90–100 ml/kg in the preterm compared to 60–70 ml/kg in adults [25]. However, when infant weight is considered in these calculations, actual volumes can be viewed in a somewhat more problematic way, as Text Box 2.1 highlights.

Text Box 2.1 Practice Point: The Significance of Blood Loss During Vascular Device Insertion

A 1 ml blood loss during vascular access insertion might represent a 2% loss of circulating blood volume in a 500 g infant.

For a 70 kg adult person, a blood loss of around 100 ml would represent an equivalent percentage loss, clearly not something that regularly features during adult vascular access procedures.

Consequently, it is essential to be mindful of accumulative blood losses.

- During blood sampling.
- During repeated attempts at obtaining vascular access.
- Failing to adequately control bleeding and prevent bruising.

Having limited circulatory volume reserves, greater blood viscosity, and immature renal functionality for regulating and conserving body fluids coupled with over-zealous or inadequate fluid infusion management can impact haemodynamic stability and the ease of obtaining vascular access in NICU infants. Careful attention to ensuring appropriate fluid balance and close monitoring of infused fluids to avoid hypo- and hypervolemia ensure optimal vasculature accessibility during insertion procedures.

2.3.2 Neonatal Physiology

2.3.2.1 Birth Transitions

Preterm infants are physiologically unready for birth and much of the research and practice attention has been focused in overcoming these constraints. Early concerns were about improving survival and completing the many gaps in our understanding of neonatal pathophysiology [8, 9]. Historically, the provision of organised hospital care for newborns, especially those born early is a relatively recent phenomenon [8, 9]. New ways of working and the clinical application of better understandings of newborn physiology and pathophysiology combined with technological developments contributed to marked decline in mortality and to the recognition of neonatology as a distinct medical speciality [6, 7, 9]. With the benefit of retrospective vision, however, not all developments were entirely positive.

One example: the professionalisation of newborn care and concerns over infection transmission resulted in the physical separation of infants from their parents in different hospital locations. This factor is widely regarded as contributing to the enduring feelings of loss and alienation reported by parents in earlier neonatal parenthood studies (e.g., [26–29]). Whilst physical separation of parents from their infants still exists in many NICUs, there are some innovative NICU designs that ensure continuity of parent–infant contact and avoid separation. Concerns over the gaps in support for parents and a desire to promote greater involvement have become influential drivers for the delivery of more developmental sensitive care.

Newborn physiology is unique in many ways and can perhaps be best considered as transitionary between that of the foetus and the older child. Some physiological changes are rapidly taking place over minutes, like those happening during the circulatory and respiratory transitions immediately after birth. These include those accompanying the onset of breathing air (lung fluid clearance, changes in pulmonary and cardiovascular/haemodynamic dynamics) and the remodelling and functional closure of cardiovascular blood flow shunts (FO, DV, DA, UAs, and UV) [30, 31]. These changes to the foetal circulation enables the transition from placental to respiratory system driven gaseous exchange. These are accompanied by further organ system adaptions to extra uterine life taking place over subsequent days, weeks, months, and years. One example is the change over from the dominance of foetal haemoglobin (HBF) to adult type (HBA) over the subsequent 6 months, affecting oxygen transport systems.

Organ systems mature differentially along non-linear trajectories. For some systems, the trigger to rapidly advance maturation (compared to the pace if birth had not occurred) is exposure to the post-birth environment. Notably affected by birth are skin maturation and metabolic/nutritional processes, including the induction of gut enzymes necessary for enteral digestion. Infants born preterm are physiologically unready for birth. These infants encounter difficulties during postnatal adaption due to immature organ systems and their differential maturation rates post-birth. Of relevance to vascular access are the post-birth developments of the integumentary and immune systems physiology and anatomy and their consequences for effective infection prevention.

2.3.2.2 Skin Development and Maturation

The skin in full term infants, whilst sufficiently mature to respond to the usual demands of postnatal barrier function, is underdeveloped at birth [32]. Post-birth, the skin undergoes a rapid period of changes in anatomy and physiology that continues for several years. Specifically, these include establishment of a protective skin microbiome, alterations in hydration, surface acidity, transepidermal water loss regulation, and immunology [33–37]. This means that term born infant skin is vulnerable to harm, sensitisation, irritation, and adverse alterations in skin barrier function due to healthcare provider and parent choices and actions. A situation that research suggests is made more acute by the effects of prematurity on skin maturation process in combination with exposure to clinical procedures and practices in NICUs [38–40].

The implications of infant skin condition at birth, its natural postnatal development, and the effects of gestation at birth on these processes, avoiding or managing existing skin damage and the like are clear for vascular access. Figure 2.1 illustrates some of the common concerns of skin management and prevention of harm research seen in the neonatal literature.

Some of these considerations feature prominently in discussions around neonatal vascular access and will be explored in more detail in Chaps. 5, 6 and 7, concerned with the insertion, use, and aftercare of vascular access devices.

2.3.2.3 Immune Development and Maturation

Preterm infants are essentially born immunocompromised, and this state can last into early childhood [41]. This situation is due to many factors including those listed in Text Box 2.2 [41–45]. Taken together, all these factors interplay and compromise the infant's ability to react to infective challenges. According to evidence and commentary, these early immune system vulnerabilities can contribute to the spectrum of cognitive, behavioural, mental health, and physiological adversities seen in children, adolescents, and adults born preterm [46–48].

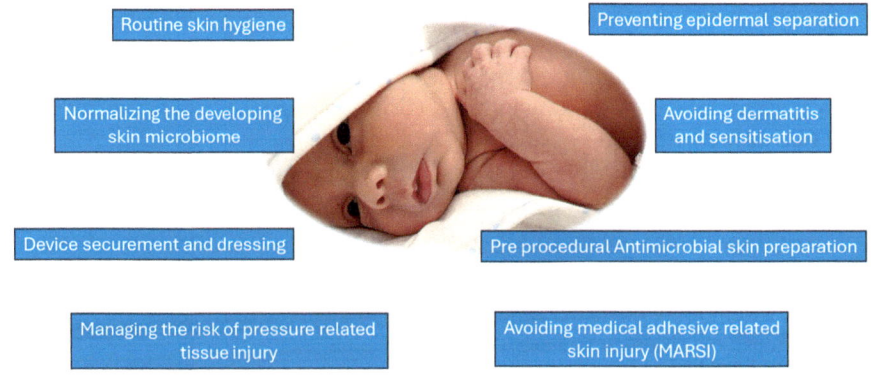

Fig. 2.1 Common management and prevention of harm concerns in neonatal skin research

Maturation of the immune system after birth progresses along complex pathways which are not entirely predictable. The composition and number of white blood cells can be mapped according to gestation and age post-birth, suggesting discrete developmental phases [49]. One study reported by Hibbert and colleagues [50] found that changes in leucocyte count and population composition persisted for up to a month after the onset and treatment of late onset sepsis in a group of preterm infants. Leucocyte counts were not only lower but had a greater preponderance of immature granulocytes. They observed that the change in leucocyte populations supports the interpretation of sepsis-induced immune suppression. There are implications of this finding for infants requiring treatment for infection with vascular access therapy. These infants remain vulnerable to repeated episodes of infection for some considerable time after successful treatment and apparent return to health. This risk should be factored into infection prevention practice and infant clinical management plans.

Other components of the immune system are less predictable. One example is the inflammatory response which is usually triggered by an infective challenge. However, in preterm infants, biomarkers of systemic inflammation are often elevated in the absence of infection [51]. The cause of this elevation is thought to be partly related to oxidative stresses. Stresses are moderated by the use of supplemental oxygen, mechanical ventilation, and parenteral nutrition. Oxidative stress and dysregulation of the inflammatory response play a role in several important morbidities and organs dysfunctions related to prematurity, including necrotising enterocolitis and bronchopulmonary dysplasia. It is reasoned that even brief periods of oxidative stress can harmful, hence the current resuscitative guidance to use air or titrate oxygen delivery according to patient need [52]. Although not straightforward nor fully understood, oxidative stress can also be induced by injury, infection, and pain experiences, matters of direct relevance to nurses involved in neonatal vascular access.

Text Box 2.2 Practice Point: Factors Affecting the Immune Status in Newborn Infants

Nurses need to be mindful of factors contributing to immature immune status in preterm infants undergoing skin breaking procedures. During patient assessment and care planning, consider the impacts of:

Underdeveloped skin barrier function
Low levels of donated maternal immunoglobulins due to curtailed pregnancy
Limited adaptive immune response capacity
Due to immune cells still undergoing ontogenesis
Unbalanced or deranged gut and skin microbiome colonisation
Exposure to repeated invasive procedures and attendant risks
The number of previous skin breaking or invasive procedures
Oxidative stress

Patient and environmental risks for hospital onset bacteraemia or fungemia (hob) and hospital-acquired infections (HAI).

In general, for those born preterm, the maturation and integration of physiological systems lag that of infants born at term gestation and can be further retarded by the pathological problems of prematurity and medical interventions intended to save lives. Doing this whilst simultaneously attempting to promote normal physiological (e.g., establishing normal skin and intestinal flora) and developmental trajectories and mitigate unintended and undesired effects is not straightforward.

The indivisible nature of human physiological, anatomical function, behavioural and developmental processes confirms the need to account for these interrelationships in care provisions and further compounds the ethics of adopting a more considered and holistic stance towards vascular access. Such an approach would integrate neuroprotective and developmentally appropriate treatment provisions for neonatal pathologies within everyday care practices like vascular access.

2.4   Approaches to Infection Prevention During Vascular Access

Preventing hospital onset bacteraemia or fungemia (HOB) and hospital-acquired infection (HAI) is a crucial component of neonatal vascular access. Infants in NICUs are particularly vulnerable to infection risks due to immaturity of their immune system and exposures to invasive clinical procedures. To mitigate these risks, most neonatal units have adopted strictly enforced evidence-based protocols, checklists, and care bundles for infection prevention and control based on best practice guidance (e.g., [53–56]). These documents invariably cite the need to observe robust hand hygiene practices, use personal protective equipment (PPE) based on risk assessment, and follow strict procedural steps for device insertion site preparation, insertion itself, device securement. In this book, these concerns are addressed within the relevant chapters concerning device insertion, use, and aftercare.

There is considerable divergence in local practices which partly reflects local priorities, assessments of patient related, healthcare provider, and hospital environment related risks and ideas about how best to apply the evidence-base. Whilst this situation is understandable, it has led to a confusing and at times contradictory variety of terminology and approaches to infection prevention, leading to a lack of standardisation, quality control, and the implementation of best practice [57].

The aseptic non-touch technique (ANTT®) clinical practice framework [57–59] has become a practice standard and is widely endorsed by vascular access associations and national healthcare authorities [54–57, 60]. Importantly the framework provides evidence-based guidance and a common shared terminology [60]. This evidence can be readily applied in neonatal patient care contexts and can reduce HAIs and HOBs [61, 62]. ANTT® is the infection prevention framework advocated for in this book. The choice of Standard-ANTT® or Surgical-ANTT® approach during vascular access related procedures is based on an assessment of low or high risk of performing the procedure without touching 'key parts' and is discussed in detail in the relevant Chapters.

2.5 Integrating Neuroprotective Measures and Integrating Families in Vascular Access

2.5.1 Parents' Experiences

The experiences of parents after admission of their infant to an NICU are often described as emotionally unsettling and relationally complex [26–29, 63]. These experiences can have long-lasting effects on parent mental health and well-being [63–66]. In the past, parents were essentially excluded, visitation tolerated, and if involved confined to passive roles [67]. This is no longer the case in many NICUs worldwide, and parental involvement has undergone profound changes with increasingly elevated levels of involvement and integration into the healthcare team [68–71]. In part these changes have arisen from a significant and influential body of neonatal parenthood research and parent advocacy (e.g., [26–29, 71–79]).

2.5.2 Developmentally Sensitive Care Practices

There are differing perspectives on what developmental is and is concerned with. Symington and Pinelli writing in 2002 [80] offered a pragmatic view:

a broad category of interventions designed to reduce the effects of stress on the infant in the NICU.

In contrast, Byers [81] suggested a more philosophical perspective:

a philosophy of care that requires rethinking the relationships between the infant, family, and healthcare providers. It includes a variety of activities that manage the environment and individualize the care… [81].

In recent times, both views have become increasingly mainstream and realigned within a human rights and ethical practice based perspective. In essence, contemporary developmental supportive care can be best defined as:

A philosophical driver for care delivery which involves putting systems and discrete interventions in place to deliver neonatal care at its ethical and clinical best. The overall intention is to optimise developmental outcomes (clinical, psychological, emotional, cognitive, and social), counter the adverse effects of prematurity and admission to a neonatal unit and promote positive experiences for infants, their parents and their healthcare providers.

In response, several models, frameworks, and programmes to inform and guide have been developed. Particularly influential are approaches promoted by the NIDCAP® Foundation International (https://nidcap.org) and the Brazelton Organization (https://brazelton.co.uk). Both these approaches accept the widely held notion, based upon the so-called synactive theory of development proposed by Als [82] that newborn infants can interact and participate with their environment and those around them.

The Neonatal Individualized Developmental Care Assessment Programme (NIDCAP®), the Brazelton Newborn Behavioural Observation (NBO™), and the Newborn Behavioural Assessment Scale (NBOS™) emphasise the centrality of behavioural and observational assessment, though take a slightly different before developing individualised support plans. The two organisations oversee programmes of education, training, assessment, and certification to ensure standardisation and are supported by robust programmes of scientific research and publications demonstrating their effectiveness on developmental outcomes. However, these approaches require strict protocol adherence and are resource intensive in terms of personnel and finance. Implementation across health systems lacking workforce capacity or economic resources is challenging, and some healthcare providers do not desire to follow certification routes.

Numerous models, frameworks, and programmes unaligned or consistent with NICDAP principles and aimed at supporting developmentally sensitive care exist. Table 2.1 lists some of them to illustrate the range and breadth of ideas and approaches.

These models, frameworks, and programmes [78, 79, 82–91] seek to address clinical, practice, patient safety, ethical, and parents expressed priorities. Many seek to create a more therapeutic environment in the NICU, promote greater support for involvement of families in care, encourage shared decision-making, and acknowledge the integral role of parents in the healthcare team. In support of these aims, parent-led groups and charities have become highly proactive in their advocacy for the needs of parents and their infants. For example, the March of Dimes (https://www.marchofdimes.org) in the USA, across Europe, the European Foundation for the Care of Newborn Infants (https://efcni.org), and in the UK Bliss (https://www.

Table 2.1 Models, frameworks, and programmes for the delivery of developmentally sensitive care	Neonatal Individualized Developmental Care Assessment Programme (NIDCAP®)
	Newborn Behavioural Observation (NBO™)
	Newborn Behavioural Assessment scale (NBOS™)
	The Universe of Developmental Care (UDC)
	Infant Behaviour assessment and Intervention program (IBAIP)
	Maternal-Infant transition program (MITP)
	Mother and Child Integrative Developmental Care
	Neonatal Integrative Developmental Care
	Age-appropriate care of the premature and critically ill hospitalised infant
	Core measures of age-appropriate care of the premature and critically ill hospitalised infant
	POPPY philosophy and model of care
	Wee Care Program—7 neuroprotective core measures
	Infant- and Family-Centred Developmental Care (IFCDC)
	Family-Integrated Care (FIC)

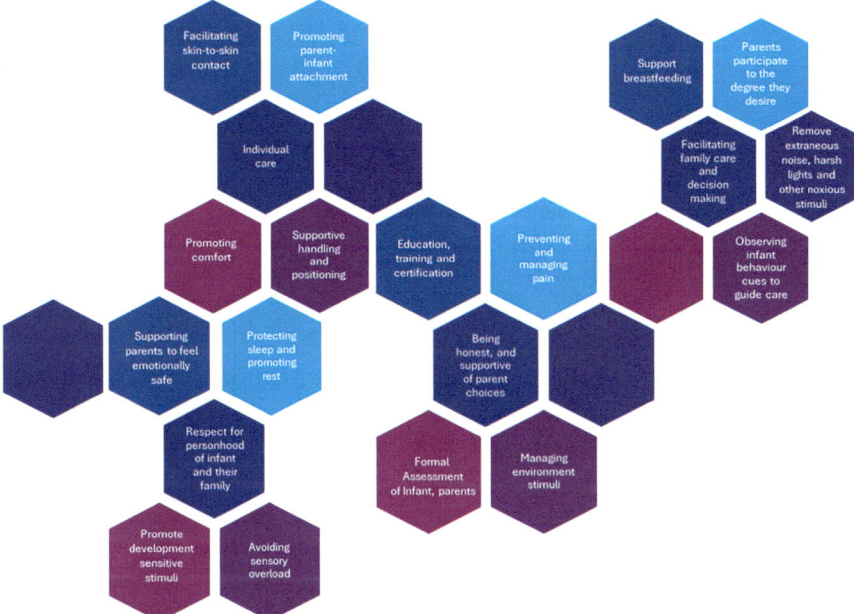

Fig. 2.2 The range of interventions promoting developmentally sensitive care

blis.org.uk). However, many of these models, frameworks, and programmes have yet to be formally evaluated in large-scale studies and have their assumptions and evidence-base tested for completeness.

Each of these models, frameworks, programmes, or ethical declarations differs in emphasising the relative importance of a range of slightly different foci of concern interventions (see Fig. 2.2). Whilst there are many areas of commonality and overlap in their interventional styles and tactics on first inspection, it is very evident that they can be readily applied to vascular access practice.

2.5.2.1 Fragmented Care

Despite the ubiquity of vascular access for newborn infants in NICUs, its practice is often seen as an 'add on' or 'a means to an end' isolated and fragmented from other facets of care. Removing these at times rigid demarcations and integrating vascular access into its proper place as an essential and fundamental part of quality care is a key motivation behind this book. Issues arising for this fragmentation are multifaceted and include those highlighted in Fig. 2.3. The subsequent chapters will explore practical examples and explanations for how developmentally sensitive interventions can be integrated within vascular access practice to defragment.

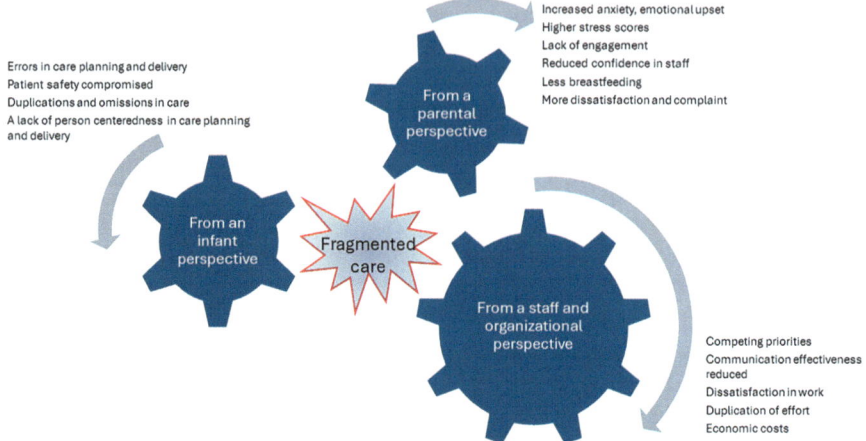

Errors in care planning and delivery
Patient safety compromised
Duplications and omissions in care
A lack of person centeredness in care planning
and delivery

Increased anxiety, emotional upset
Higher stress scores
Lack of engagement
Reduced confidence in staff
Less breastfeeding
More dissatisfaction and complaint

From a parental perspective

From an infant perspective

Fragmented care

From a staff and organizational perspective

Competing priorities
Communication effectiveness reduced
Dissatisfaction in work
Duplication of effort
Economic costs

Fig. 2.3 Issues arising from the fragmentation of care

2.6   Planning for Vascular Access Needs

Clinical management plans are a common feature in many areas of healthcare. Although the exact terminology, structure, focus, and content of these plans, quality statements, toolkits, and care pathways can vary. In some contexts, these plans operate within a specific area of patient care or legalistic framework. Examples include nurse independent and supplemental prescribing in safeguarding, the newborn infant physical examination (NIPE) programme, and end-of-life care.

In more general use, these clinical management plans are often used to set out an agreed multi-professional/multiple agency definitive plan of treatment and care for an individual named patient. Vascular access management regularly features in areas of healthcare which require safe, reliable, and uninterrupted access to the circulatory system. For example, for people who require vascular access for long-term therapies such as parenteral nutrition or renal dialysis. However, planning around vascular access is, with some exceptions, less common in many healthcare settings, engendering a more reactive response towards vascular practices. Reflecting on the vulnerabilities of infants in NICU and the intractable high rates of vascular access related complications, it can be persuadably argued that these infants could benefit from a more considered approach. Vascular access is emerging as a sub-speciality in its own right across multiple areas of healthcare and becoming more prominent within neonatal nursing. This development is supportive of efforts to take a more proactive planned approach for neonatal vascular access.

A vascular access management plan for neonates (n-VAMP) sets out a strategy for vascular access and can be broadly defined as:

> *An agreed multi-professional plan for anticipating vascular therapy needs and coordinating actions around obtaining vascular access, using it, and removing devices afterwards for a named infant.*

Such plans should ideally aim to be prospective meeting existing and anticipated therapeutic needs, preserve veins, direct the choice of the most appropriate access (device and route), anticipate issues and complications, consider parents' opinions in shared decision-making, direct to best evidence-based practices, and set the boundaries for vascular access practice amongst junior nurses and healthcare providers.

Text Box 2.3 Practice Point: Reflecting on n-VAMP Implementation in Clinical Settings

Consider a scenario where an infant in the NICU requires long-term vascular access.

How would you approach the creation of a vascular access management plan for this infant to meet their immediate and longer term needs?

Reflect on any specific considerations (such as individual vulnerabilities, potential complications, and parental input) that you would need to consider.

- How might you prioritise these considerations?
- In your experience, how might the implementation of an n-VAMP impact the outcomes for infants requiring vascular access?
- What challenges might arise in your practice setting, and how could these be mitigated?

2.6.1 Constructing an n-VAMP

Any plans for vascular access must be dynamic and reviewed in the light of changing situations and information. This periodic reappraisal relies on input from the multi-professional team and parents and builds into the n-VAMP cyclical processes that ensure that individual infant needs remain foundational to care and management decisions and practices.

One approach for constructing an n-VAMP is to use a series of information gathering, decision-making, and practice directing building blocks. This section proposes one example to illustrate this conceptual approach. Figure 2.4 illustrates this approach for the phased construction of an n-VAMP. There are three primary phases, accompanied by integral sub-phases, which are used in a sequential and cyclical process to direct the production of an individualised plan. The three phases are described as follows.

2.6.1.1 Preliminary Considerations and Assessments

Determining the indication for infusion therapy based on:

- Reviewing infant medical history
- Assessing the degree of urgency, infant clinical stability or deteriorating, impact of behavioural cues and ability to tolerate procedure
- Factoring in parents' opinions

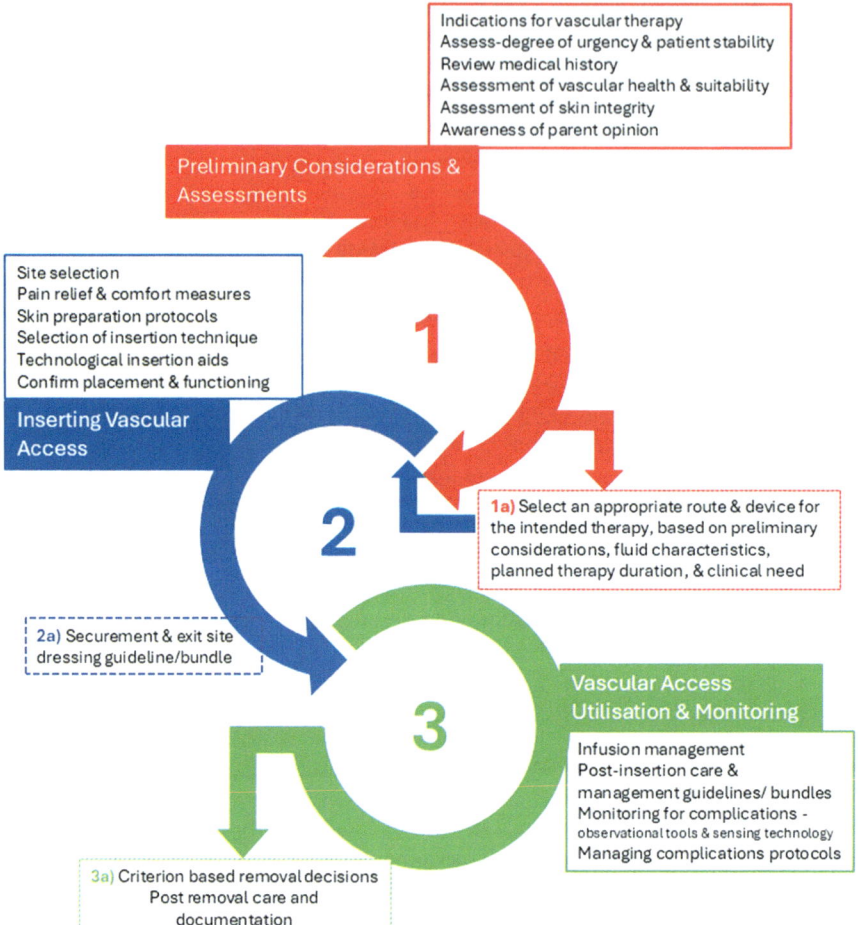

Fig. 2.4 Building a neonatal vascular access management plan

- Undertaking systematic evaluations of skin and vascular health and suitability and other risk factors for complications (e.g., prematurity, low birth weight, existing pathology).

Decision-Making Sub-phase
Deciding upon an appropriate device and route (peripheral/central) based on:

- Evaluating characteristics of the fluids to be infused
- Requirements for blood sampling or haemodynamic monitoring
- Anticipating therapy duration and need for future vascular access (e.g., <72 h, >5 days, >14 days)
- Balancing evaluation of potential risks and benefits from choosing different devices and routes

- Examining previous history of vascular access, difficulties (difficult intravenous access, DIVA), and complications.

2.6.1.2 Inserting Vascular Access

Obtaining vascular access safely and effectively based on:

- Site selecting, applying appropriate skin disinfection and non-touch antiseptic technique protocols and care bundles
- Providing effective comfort promoting and pain relief measures
- Using technological aids for vascular assessment to assist with site selection and insertion
- Insertion technique determined by device and route choice
- Confirming correct device placement and functioning.

Decision-Making Sub-phase

Deciding on appropriate device securement and exit site protection based on:

- Implementing evidence-based device securement and exit site protective dressing guidelines and care bundles.

2.6.1.3 Vascular Access Utilisation and Monitoring

Safely using vascular access based on:

- Post-insertion care and management of the device guidelines and care bundles.
- Infusion management—safe use of infusion pumps, regular review, and adjustment as needed.
- Monitoring for and managing complications—observation, technological aids, and protocols.

Decision-Making Sub-phase

Criterion-based decisions as to when to discontinue therapy and remove the device based on:

- Factoring in clinical and therapy needs, infant well-being, and presence/risk of complications.
- Addressing post-removal care needs and documentation, team debriefing, audit, and quality reporting.

Ideas and evidence about the contents of the individual building blocks within the n-VAMP continues to emerge and many of these aspects will be considered in subsequent chapters of this book. Considerable elements of vascular access can be protocolised and predicted, which is a key strength of care bundles and treatment algorithms. Planning frameworks such as proposed here can accommodate individual variation and need whilst continuing to ensure that practice remains evidence driven. Despite this, one question that repeatedly rises to the fore in everyday practice is: 'In anticipation of this situation what device should be used?' Answering this question is challenging, often there is no single correct answer but several answers. The most comprehensive answer is to use a device that has the lowest risk of complications, meets therapy needs, ensures infant well-being, and is acceptable to healthcare providers and parents alike, a tall order to fulfil.

2.6.2 Factors to Consider When Deciding on Which Intravenous Access Device

The selection of the most appropriate vascular access device, in any given circumstances is one of the key strategies in modifying the risk of harm. However, choice in paediatrics is limited [92, 93]. Fernández-Fernández et al. [94] in a systematic review observed considerable variation in opinion about what was considered 'optimal'. This they attributed to interpersonal and cultural factors. However, less variation was noted in settings which had established specialised vascular access management teams. This finding might be due to having a shared vision, standardised education, training, and guidelines, as well as greater teamworking reported by other studies looking into vascular teams [95–97], Establishing multi-professional generalist and specialist vascular access team is generally associated with better patient outcomes [56, 98].

Blood vessel selection and the route for vascular access (peripheral or central blood vessels) in neonates is a complex undertaking that requires high levels of reasoning. Choices are primarily driven by current clinical need and not anticipating future needs. Several consensus statements and algorithms have been developed to help inform practice decisions concern device selection [93, 99–102]. Some (e.g., [93, 102]) argue that current versions lack comprehensive consideration of neonatal vascular access needs; this they attribute to:

- Differing use of vascular access terminology.
- Not differentiating between the needs of term, moderately preterm and extremely preterm infants and infants of different age post-birth.
- Not differentiating between the needs of haemodynamically stable, unstable infants or those in emergency situations.
- Applying different weightings to the importances of factors known to affect decisions about devices and blood vessel suitability.
- Differing interpretations of what is an appropriate indication for using a device or approach.
- Incomplete integration of newer approaches and technologies into device selection (e.g., pre-procedural systematic assessment of vasculature using ultrasound).

Whilst many of these observations are valid, designing a process to guide decision-making that captures the complexity of every possible vascular access decision and ensures that it remains contemporaneous as new evidence emerges is fraught with considerable difficulties. Fig. 2.5 sets out the extensive range of

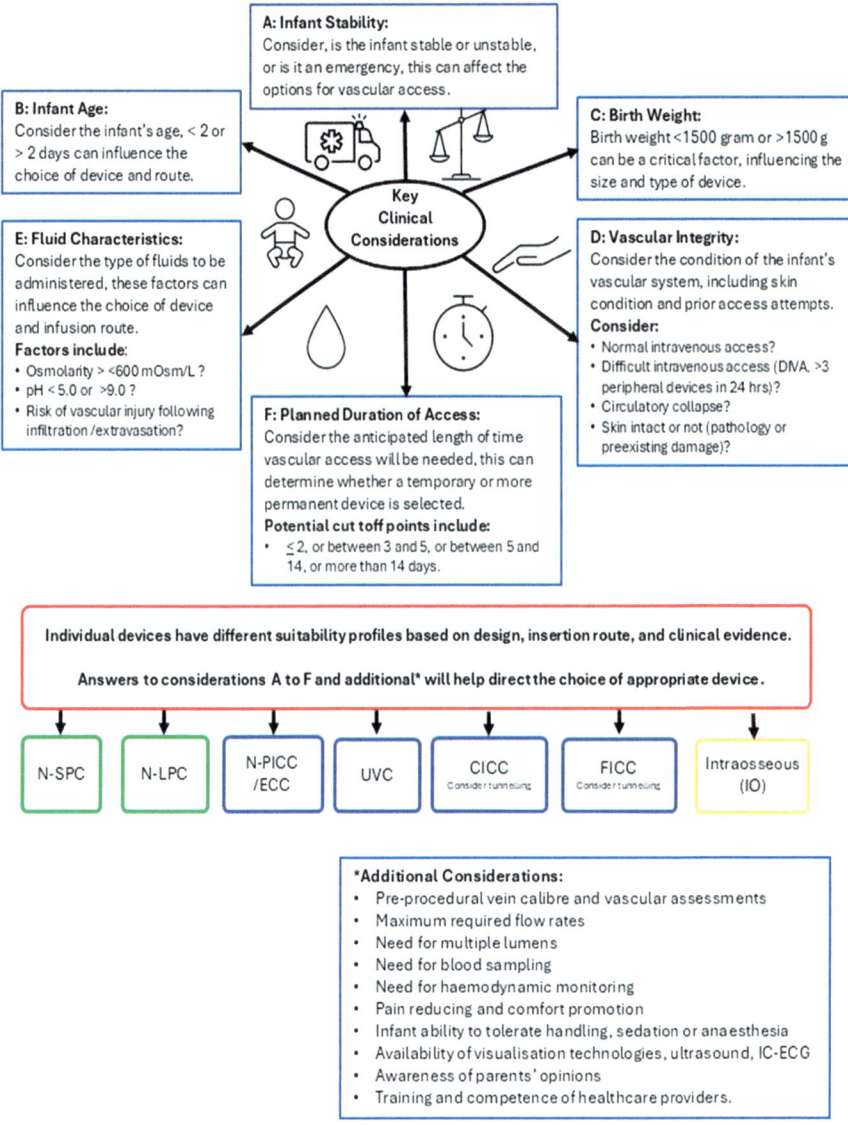

Fig. 2.5 Factors to consider when designing an intravenous access device selection algorithm

considerations that need to be accounted for when designing a neonatal vascular access device and route algorithm as an informative guide to prompt further debate, reflection, and consideration of what informs individual nurses' choices around vascular access device.

In summary, a key benefit of developing an n-VAMP is that it offers a new perspective and brings together for consideration all the complexities that can influence the safety and successful delivery of vascular therapies into one framework. These plans can be used to support the dissemination of newer approaches to vascular access and can be readily unified within overall multidisciplinary clinical management of sick and preterm infants in NICUs. A strategic and dynamic plan around vascular access can ensure the continuation of infant centeredness into this key area of care and eliminate nurse, healthcare provider, or organisational expediencies around vascular access practice. Key steps in devising a meaningful n-VAMP include assessment, device (and route) selection, implementation of best evidence-based practices, monitoring for complications (and their effective treatment), and making informed decisions about removal and discontinuation. Incorporating parent's views and preferences into planning can engender greater family integration in overall care activities [91].

2.7   Terminologies Used in This Book

2.7.1   Vascular Access Devices

The terminology around neonatal vascular access has evolved to reflect changes in knowledge, device use, and the increased range of design options available. However, there is lag between the words used in everyday practice in different regional and international neonatal care settings and those used in research, manufacture, and education. Whilst the words are often understood within their local context, their use beyond can create confusion and uncertainty. In this book, we use the descriptive terms outlined in Table 2.2 to describe neonatal vascular access catheters. These terms align with international guidelines and more recent position statements by professional vascular access representative organisations [92, 103, 104] and are further described within their relevant chapters.

Table 2.2 A typology of neonatal vascular access devices

Device name	Abbreviation
Peripheral venous access devices	PVAD
Neonatal-short peripheral catheter—Less than 2 cm long	n-SPC
Neonatal-long peripheral catheter—Between 2 cm and 6 cm long	n-LPC
Central venous access devices	CVAD
Umbilical venous catheter	UVC
Neonatal-peripherally inserted central catheter or Epicutaneo-cava catheter	n-PICC or ECC
Central inserted central catheter	CICC
Femoral inserted central catheter	FICC
Intra-arterial catheters Further classified by the artery inserted into, e.g., femoral artery, radial artery, or umbilical artery (UAC)	IAC
Intraosseous device	IO

2.8   Concluding Remarks

In summary, this chapter has laid the foundation for essential knowledge by providing an overview of some general considerations associated with managing neonatal vascular access and the need for proactive planning around securing, using, and managing this access using a conceptual planning framework (a n-VAMP). This knowledge will underpin the subsequent chapters.

Preterm birth, illness at birth, and the effects of NICU admission and associated clinical interventions can interfere with post-birth transitions and developmental maturation of organ systems in complex and not entirely predictable ways. Navigating these complexities, treating neonatal pathologies whilst simultaneously supporting normal post-birth transitions, autoregulation, and development are key challenges in neonatology. Ideas about how best to mitigate the developmental consequences of preterm birth, illness, NICU admission, and support families during their time on the NICU become established in practice and expressed in several overlapping models of care delivery. Common concepts include implementing neuroprotective measures and integrating care practices within families. As a result, in more recent decades, parents have become increasingly recognised as integral members of the healthcare team and consequently their roles have evolved and become increasingly proactive in many aspects of care for their infant. However, parental involvement in some areas of care, like vascular access is less universally developed and opportunities exist to improve this situation.

> **Key Points**
> - Newborn infants have many unique features due to their distinctive anatomy and physiology and post-birth adaptive processes.
> - Knowledge about infant anatomical and physiological developmental transitions post-birth is foundational for safe practice.
> - Neonatal vascular access requires special considerations due to the challenges posed by prematurity.
> - Due to inherent vulnerabilities for infection risk assessment and strict adherence to infection, prevention measures and aseptic technique are essential.
> - Neonatal vascular access procedures are often considered in isolation from other essential aspects of care, and this leads to fragmentation of care.
> - Developmental models, frameworks, and programmes of care offer the opportunity to better integrate vascular access with wider care concerns in developmentally sensitive and responsive ways.
> - Proactive planning using systematic frameworks (e.g., n-VAMP) around the management of neonatal vascular access can help justify decisions and choices, and evidence how the philosophical stance of infant centeredness is embedded in practice.
> - The terminology around neonatal vascular access devices lacks consensus, but this situation is changing.

Reflective Activity: Experiences of Neonatal Vascular Access
Read the following case related to an episode of vascular access and consider your responses to the reflective questions at the end.

Monica is a 3-day-old infant born preterm in good health weighing 1.02 kg. Monica has been prescribed intravenous (IV) antibiotic therapy for suspected sepsis based on clinical presentation. It was emphasised to the bedside nurse that this therapy should begin as soon as possible. Monica does not currently have a peripheral vascular access device (PVAD) in situ and is a little unsettled. As is usual in the unit, the bedside nurse is primarily responsible for inserting the PVAD. However, despite multiple attempts using four different 22-gauge short peripheral catheter (n-SPC) devices, the nurse is unable to obtain access even when attempting to insert in the right basilic vein. The nurse attributes this to the fragility of Monica's veins rather than any other factors and seeks assistance from a vascular access specialist colleague. This colleague successfully inserts a 24-gauge n-SPC using an ultrasound-guided technique with assistance of the bedside nurse holding and comforting Monica without complication. Monica was able to commence antibiotic therapy without undue delay.

Considering the above case, reflect on your answers to the following questions:

1. How could the bedside nurse have done things differently to improve the likelihood of first-attempt successful PVAD insertion?
   (a) Consider what factors of neonatal anatomy and behaviour did the nurse fail to consider that would have impacted on the difficulty of finding a suitable vein and inserting the device?
2. If you were the specialist nurse, how would you debrief the bedside nurse to ensure that they learnt from this experience?
   (a) Consider what key learning points around vein identification and use, device selection choices, acceptable numbers of attempts before seeking assistance and meeting unmet needs of Monica during these insertion attempts you would like to convey.

References

1. Cosnett JE. The origins of intravenous fluid therapy. Lancet. 1989;1(8641):768–71. https://doi.org/10.1016/s0140-6736(89)92583-x.
2. Sette P, Dorizzi RM, Azzini AM. Vascular access: an historical perspective from Sir William Harvey to the 1956 Nobel Prize to André F. Cournand, Werner Forssmann, and Dickinson W. Richards. J Vasc Access. 2012;13(2):137–44. https://doi.org/10.5301/jva.5000018.
3. Millam D. The history of intravenous therapy. J Intraven Nurs. 1996;19(1):5–14.
4. Ball C. The early development of intravenous apparatus. Anaesth Intensive Care. 2006;34(S1):22–6.

5. Rivera AM, Strauss KW, Van Zundert A, Mortier E. The history of peripheral intravenous catheters: how little plastic tubes revolutionized medicine. Acta Anaesth Belg. 2005;56(3):271–82.

6. Henderson B. The history of neonatal care: a snapshot of its birth as a speciality. J Neonat Nurs. 2001;7(6):190–4.

7. Philip A. The evolution of neonatology. Pediatr Res. 2005;58(4):799–815. https://doi.org/10.1203/01.PDR.0000151693.46655.6.

8. Dunn PM. Erratum to: the birth of perinatal medicine in the United Kingdom. Sem Fetal Neonatal Med. 2007;11(6):386–97. Sem Fetal Neonat Med. 2007;12(3):226–38

9. Christie DA, Tansey EM, editors. Welcome witness to twentieth century medicine: origins of neonatal intensive care in the UK (9). London: Welcome Trust Centre at University College; 2001. https://wellcomecollection.org/works/znbxa5qs. Accessed 12 August 2024

10. Southorn PA, Narr BJ. The Massa or Rochester plastic needle. Mayo Clin Proc. 2008;83(10):1165–7.

11. van Rens MFPT, Hugill K, Mahmah MA, Francia ALV, van Loon FHJ. Effect of peripheral intravenous catheter type and material on therapy failure in a neonatal population. J Vasc Access. 2022;24:11297298221080071. https://doi.org/10.1177/11297298221080071.

12. Stanley MD, Meister E, Fuschuber K. Infiltration during intravenous therapy in neonates: comparison of Teflon and Vialon catheters. South Med J. 1992;85(9):883–6. https://doi.org/10.1097/00007611-199209000-00006.

13. Tobin CR. The Teflon intravenous catheter: incidence of phlebitis and duration of catheter life in the neonatal patient. J Obstet Gynecol Neonat Nurs. 1988;17(1):35–42. https://doi.org/10.1111/j.1552-6909.1988.tb00412.x.

14. Kuş B, Büyükyılmaz F. Effectiveness of Vialon biomaterial versus Teflon catheters for peripheral intravenous placement: a randomized clinical trial. Jpn J Nurs Sci. 2020;17(3):e12328. https://doi.org/10.1111/jjns.12328.

15. de Lutio E. Which material and device? The choice of PICC. In: Sandrucci S, Mussa B, editors. Peripherally inserted central venous catheters. Milano: Springer; 2014. p. 7–19.

16. D'Andrea V, Prontera G, Rubortone S, Pittiruti M. Epicutaneo-cava catheters. Chapter 11. In: Biasucci DG, Disma NM, Pittiruti M, editors. Vascular access in neonates and children. Geneva: Springer; 2022. p. 169–88.

17. Hugill K, Van Rens M. Inserting central lines via the peripheral circulation in neonates. Brit J Nurs. 2020;29(19):S12–8. https://doi.org/10.12968/bjon.2020.29.19.S12.

18. van Rens MFPT, Hugill K, van den Lee R, Francia ALV, van Loon FHJ, Bayoumi MAA. Comparing conventional and modified Seldinger technique using a micro insertion kit for PICC placement in neonates: a retrospective cohort study. Front Pediatr. 2024;12:1395395. https://doi.org/10.3389/fped.2024.1395395.

19. Bayoumi MAA, van Rens MFPT, Chandra P, Masry A, D'Souza S, Khalil AM, et al. Does the antimicrobial-impregnated peripherally inserted central catheter decrease the CLABSI rate in neonates? Results from a retrospective cohort study. Front Pediatr. 2022;10:1012800. https://doi.org/10.3389/fped.2022.1012800.

20. Gilbert R, Brown M, Rainford N, Donohue C, Fraser C, Sinha A, et al. Antimicrobial-impregnated central venous catheters for prevention of neonatal bloodstream infection (PREVAIL): an open-label, parallel-group, pragmatic, randomised controlled trial. Lancet Child Adolesc Health. 2019;3(6):381–90. https://doi.org/10.1016/S2352-4642(19)30114-2.

21. van Rens MFPT, Hugill K, Mahmah MA, Bayoumi M, Francia ALV, Garcia KLP, et al. Evaluation of unmodifiable and potentially modifiable factors affecting peripheral intravenous device-related complications in neonates: a retrospective observational study. BMJ Open. 2021;11(9):e047788. https://doi.org/10.1136/bmjopen-2020-047788.

22. Legemaat M, Carr PJ, van Rens MFPT, Van Dijk M, Poslawsky IE, van den Hoogen A. Peripheral intravenous cannulation: complication rates in the neonatal population: a multicenter observational study. J Vasc Access. 2016;17(4):360–5. https://doi.org/10.5301/jva.5000558.

23. Indarwati F, Mathew S, Munday J, Keogh S. Incidence of peripheral intravenous catheter failure and complications in paediatric patients: systematic review and meta analysis. Int J Nurs Stud. 2020;102:103488. https://doi.org/10.1016/J.IJNURSTU.2019.103488.
24. Atay S, Sen S, Cukurlu D. Incidence of infiltration/extravasation in newborns using peripheral venous catheter and affecting factors. Rev Esc Enferm USP. 2018;52:e03360. https://doi.org/10.1590/S1980-220X2017040103360.
25. Roseff SDS, Luban NLC, Manno CS. Guidelines for assessing appropriateness of pediatric transfusion. Transfusion. 2002;42(11):1398–413. https://doi.org/10.1046/j.1537-2995.2002.00208.x.
26. Jackson K, Ternestedt BM, Schollin J. From alienation to familiarity: experiences of mothers and fathers of preterm infants. J Adv Nurs. 2003;43(2):120–9. https://doi.org/10.1046/j.1365-2648.2003.02686.x.
27. Davis L, Edwards H, Mohay H, Wollin J. The impact of very premature birth on the psychological health of mothers. Early Human Dev. 2003;73(1–2):61–70.
28. Hugill K, Letherby G, Reid T, Lavender T. Experiences of fathers shortly after the birth of their preterm infants. J Obstet Gynecol Neonat Nurs. 2013;42(6):655–63. https://doi.org/10.1111/1552-6909.12256.
29. Spinelli M, Frigerio A, Montali L, Fasolo M, Spada MS, Mangili G. 'I still have difficulties feeling like a mother': the transition to motherhood of preterm infants' mothers. Psychol Health. 2016;31(2):184–204. https://doi.org/10.1080/08870446.2015.1088015.
30. Hugill K, Meredith D. The road to life. Neonatal transitions to extra-uterine life. Practising Midwife. 2017;20(6):10–4.
31. Morton SU, Brodsky D. Fetal physiology and the transition to extrauterine life. Clin Perinatol. 2016;43(3):395–407. https://doi.org/10.1016/j.clp.2016.04.001.
32. Visscher MO, Carr AN, Winget J, Huggins T, Bascom CC, Isfort R, et al. Biomarkers of neonatal skin barrier adaptation reveal substantial differences compared to adult skin. Pediatr Res. 2021;89(5):1208–15. https://doi.org/10.1038/s41390-020-1035-y.
33. Fluhr JW, Darlenski R, Lachmann N, Baudouin C, Msika P, De Belilovsky C, et al. Infant epidermal skin physiology: adaptation after birth. Br J Dermatol. 2012;166(3):483–90. https://doi.org/10.1111/j.1365-2133.2011.10659.x.
34. Townsend EC, Kalan LR. The dynamic balance of the skin microbiome across the lifespan. Biochem Soc Trans. 2023;51(1):71–86. https://doi.org/10.1042/BST20220216.
35. Trompette A, Ubags ND. Skin barrier immunology from early life to adulthood. Mucosal Immunol. 2023;16(2):194–207. https://doi.org/10.1016/j.mucimm.2023.02.005.
36. Harrison IS, Monir RL, Neu J, Schoch JJ. Neonatal sepsis and the skin microbiome. J Perinatol. 2022;42(11):1429–33. https://doi.org/10.1038/s41372-022-01451-0.
37. Zhang C, Merana GR, Harris-Tryon T, Scharschmidt TC. Skin immunity: dissecting the complex biology of our body's outer barrier. Mucosal Immunol. 2022;15(4):551–61. https://doi.org/10.1038/s41385-022-00505-y.
38. Oranges T, Dini V, Romanelli M. Skin physiology of the neonate and infant: clinical implications. Adv Wound Care (New Rochelle). 2015;4(10):587–95. https://doi.org/10.1089/wound.2015.0642.
39. Visscher MO, Carr AN, Narendran V. Premature infant skin barrier maturation: status at full-term corrected age. J Perinatol. 2021;41(2):232–9. https://doi.org/10.1038/s41372-020-0704-3.
40. Agren J, Sjörs G, Sedin G. Transepidermal water loss in infants born at 24 and 25 weeks of gestation. Acta Paediatr. 1998;87(11):1185–90. https://doi.org/10.1080/080352598750031194.
41. Melville JM, Moss TJ. The immune consequences of preterm birth. Front Neurosci. 2013;7:79. https://doi.org/10.3389/fnins.2013.00079.
42. Strunk T, Currie A, Richmond P, Simmer K, Burgner D. Innate immunity in human newborn infants: prematurity means more than immaturity. J Matern Fetal Neonat Med. 2011;24(1):25–31. https://doi.org/10.3109/14767058.2010.482605.

43. Nunez N, Réot L, Menu E. Neonatal immune system ontogeny: the role of maternal micro-biota and associated factors. How might the non-human primate model enlighten the path? Vaccines (Basel). 2021;9(6):584. https://doi.org/10.3390/vaccines9060584.
44. Qazi KR, Bach Jensen G, van der Heiden M, Björkander S, Holmlund U, Haileselassie Y, et al. Extremely preterm infants have significant alterations in their conventional T cell compartment during the first weeks of life. J Immunol. 2020;204(1):68–77. https://doi.org/10.4049/jimmunol.1900941.
45. Henderickx JGE, Zwittink RD, Renes IB, van Lingen RA, van Zoeren-Grobben D, et al. Maturation of the preterm gastrointestinal tract can be defined by host and microbial mark-ers for digestion and barrier defence. Sci Rep. 2021;11:2808. https://doi.org/10.1038/s41598-021-92222-y.
46. Luu TM, Rehman Mian MO, Nuyt AM. Long-term impact of preterm birth: neurodevel-opmental and physical health outcomes. Clin Perinatol. 2017;44(2):305–14. https://doi.org/10.1016/j.clp.2017.01.003.
47. Crump C. An overview of adult health outcomes after preterm birth. Early Hum Dev. 2020;150:105187. https://doi.org/10.1016/j.earlhumdev.2020.105187.
48. Humberg A, Fortmann I, Siller B, Kopp MV, Herting E, Göpel W, et al. Preterm birth and sustained inflammation: consequences for the neonate. Semin Immunopathol. 2020;42(4):451–68. https://doi.org/10.1007/s00281-020-00803-2.
49. Walker JC, Smolders MA, Gemen EF, Antonius TA, Leuvenink J, de Vries E. Development of lymphocyte subpopulations in preterm infants. Scand J Immunol. 2011;73(1):53–8. https://doi.org/10.1111/j.1365-3083.2010.02473.x.
50. Hibbert J, Strunk T, Nathan E, Prosser A, Doherty D, Simmer K, et al. Composition of early life leukocyte populations in preterm infants with and without late-onset sepsis. PLoS One. 2022;17(3):e0264768. https://doi.org/10.1371/journal.pone.0264768.
51. Chang BA, Huang Q, Quan J, Chau V, Ladd M, Kwan E, et al. Early inflammation in the absence of overt infection in preterm neonates exposed to intensive care. Cytokine. 2011;56(3):621–6. https://doi.org/10.1016/j.cyto.2011.08.028.
52. Madar J, Roehr CR, Ainsworth S, Ersdal H, Morley C, Rüdiger M, et al. European Resuscitation Council guidelines 2021: newborn resuscitation and support of transition of infants at birth. Resuscitation. 2021;161:291–326. https://doi.org/10.1016/j.resuscitation.2021.02.014.
53. Glowicz JB, Landon E, Sickbert-Bennett EE, Aiello AE, deKay K, Hoffmann KK, et al. SHEA/IDSA/APIC practice recommendation: strategies to prevent healthcare-associated infections through hand hygiene: 2022 update. Infect Control Hosp Epidemiol. 2023;44(3):355–76. https://doi.org/10.1017/ice.2022.304.
54. Centers for Disease Control and Prevention (CDC). CDC's core infection prevention and con-trol practices for safe healthcare delivery in all settings. (29 November 2022). https://www.cdc.gov/infectioncontrol/guidelines/core-practices/index.html. Accessed 12 August 2024.
55. National Health Service (NHS) England. National infection prevention and control manual for England, V2.4. London: NHS England; 2023.
56. Nickel B, Gorski L, Kleidon T, Kyes A, DeVries M, Keogh S, et al. Infusion therapy standards of practice. 9th ed. J Inf Nurs. 2024;47(1S):S1–285. https://doi.org/10.1097/NAN.0000000000000532.
57. Rowley S, Clare S. Guidance document. Standardizing the critical clinical competency of aseptic, sterile, and clean techniques with a single international standard: aseptic non touch technique (ANTT®). Mount Royal: Association for Vascular Access; 2019. https://cdn.ymaws.com/www.avainfo.org/resource/resmgr/files/position_statements/ANTT.pdf. Accessed 12 August 2024
58. Rowley S, Clare S, MacQueen S, Molyneux R. ANTT® v2: an updated practice framework for aseptic technique. Brit J Nurs. 2010;19:S5–11.
59. ANTT® procedure guidelines. https://www.antt.org/antt-procedure-guidelines.html. Accessed 12 August 2024.
60. Clare S, Rowley S. Implementing the aseptic non touch technique (ANTT®) clini-cal practice framework for aseptic technique: a pragmatic evaluation using a mixed

methods approach in two London hospitals. J Infect Prev. 2018;19(1):6–15. https://doi. org/10.1177/1757177417720996.

61. Khurana S, Saini SS, Sundaram V, Dutta S, Kumar P. Reducing healthcare-associated infections in neonates by standardizing and improving compliance to aseptic non-touch techniques: a quality improvement approach. Indian Pediatr. 2018;55(9):748–52.

62. Shettigar S, Somasekhara Aradhya A, Ramappa S, Reddy V, Venkatagiri P. Reducing healthcare-associated infections by improving compliance to aseptic non-touch technique in intravenous line maintenance: a quality improvement approach. BMJ Open Qual. 2021;10:e001394. https://doi.org/10.1136/bmjoq-2021-001394.

63. Lakshmanan A, Agni M, Lieu T, Fleegler E, Kipke M, Friedlich PS, et al. The impact of preterm birth <37 weeks on parents and families: a cross-sectional study in the 2 years after discharge from the neonatal intensive care unit. Health Qual Life Outcomes. 2017;15(1):38. https://doi.org/10.1186/s12955-017-0602-3.

64. Schecter R, Pham T, Hua A, Spinazzola R, Sonnenklar J, Li D, et al. Prevalence and longevity of PTSD symptoms among parents of NICU infants analyzed across gestational age categories. Clin Pediatr (Phila). 2020;59(2):163–9. https://doi.org/10.1177/0009922819892046.

65. McKeown L, Burke K, Cobham VE, Kimball H, Foxcroft K, Callaway L. The prevalence of PTSD of mothers and fathers of high-risk infants admitted to NICU: a systematic review. Clin Child Fam Psychol Rev. 2023;26(1):33–49. https://doi.org/10.1007/s10567-022-00421-4.

66. Voulgaridou A, Paliouras D, Defteros S, Skarentzos K, Tsergoula E, Miltsakaki I, et al. Hospitalization in neonatal intensive care unit: parental anxiety and satisfaction. Pan Afr Med J. 2023;44:55. https://doi.org/10.11604/pamj.2023.44.55.34344.

67. Pace Parascandalo R, Hugill K. Supporting early parenting following preterm birth. In: Borg-Xuereb R, Jones J, editors. Perspectives in midwifery and parenthood. London: Springer; 2023. p. 83–94.

68. Toren O, Nirel N, Tsur Y, Lipschuetz M, Toker A. Examining professional boundaries between nurses and physicians in neonatal intensive care units. Israel J Health Policy Res. 2014;3:43. http://www.ijhpr.org/content/3/1/43

69. Celenza JF, Zayack D, Buus-Frank ME, Horbar JD. Family involvement in quality improvement: from bedside advocate to system advisor. Clinics Perinatol. 2017;44(3):553–66. https://doi.org/10.1016/j.clp.2017.05.008.

70. British Association of Perinatal medicine (BAPM). Enhancing shared decision making in neonatal care: a BAPM framework for practice. London: BAPM; 2019.

71. Balice-Bourgois C, Zumstein-Shaha M, Simonetti GD, Newman CJ. Interprofessional collaboration and involvement of parents in the management of painful procedures in newborns. Front Pediatr. 2020;8:394. https://doi.org/10.3389/fped.2020.00394.

72. Thomson G, Hall-Moran V, Axelin A, Dykes F, Flacking R. Integrating a sense of coherence into the neonatal environment. BMC Pediatr. 2013;13(84) https://doi.org/10.1186/1471-2431-13-84.

73. Petty J, Jarvis J, Thomas R. Listening to the parent voice to inform person-centred neonatal care. J Neonat Nurs. 2019;25(3):121–6. https://doi.org/10.1016/j.jnn.2019.01.005.

74. Flacking R, Lehtonen L, Thomson G, Axelin A, Ahlqvist S, Moran VH, et al. Closeness and separation in neonatal intensive care. Acta Paediatr. 2012;101(10):1032–7. https://doi.org/10.1111/j.1651-2227.2012.02787.x.

75. Carozza S, Leong V. The role of affectionate caregiver touch in early neurodevelopment and parent–infant interactional synchrony. Front Neurosci. 2021;14:613378. https://doi.org/10.3389/fnins.2020.613378.

76. Symington A, Pinelli J. Developmental care for promoting development and preventing morbidity in preterm infants. Cochrane Database Syst Rev. 2006;2006(2):CD001814. https://doi.org/10.1002/14651858.CD001814.

77. Gallagher K, Shaw C, Aladangady N, Marlow N. Parental experience of interaction with healthcare professionals during their infant's stay in the neonatal intensive care unit. Arch Dis Child Fetal Neonat Ed. 2018;103(4):F343–8. https://doi.org/10.1136/archdischild-2016-312278.

78. European Foundation for the Care of Newborn Infants (EFCNI). Infant and family-centered developmental care. European standards of care for newborn health. Munich: EFCNI; 2018. https://newborn-health-standards.org/downloads/. Accessed 12 August 2024

79. Kelly H. Putting families at the heart of their baby's care. J Neonat Nurs. 2018;24:13–6. https://doi.org/10.1016/j.jnn.2017.11.005.

80. Symington A, Pinelli JM. Distilling the evidence on developmental care: a systematic review. Adv Neonat Care. 2002;2(4):198–221. https://doi.org/10.1053/adnc.2002.34546.

81. Byers JF. Components of developmental care and the evidence for their use in the NICU. Am J Mat Child Nurs. 2003;28(3):174–80. https://doi.org/10.1097/00005721-200305000-00007.

82. Als H. Towards a synactive theory of development: promise for the assessment of infant individuality. Infant Mental Health J. 1982;3(4):229–43.

83. Westrup B. Newborn Individualized Developmental Care and Assessment Program (NIDCAP)—family-centered developmentally supportive care. Early Human Dev. 2007;83:443–9.

84. Gibbins S, Hoath S, Coughlin M, Gibbins A, Franck L. The universe of developmental care: a new conceptual model for application in the neonatal intensive care unit. Foundations Newborn Care. 2008;8(3):141–7.

85. National Association of Neonatal Nurses (NANN). Age appropriate care of the premature and critically ill hospitalized infant: guideline for practice. Glenview: NANN; 2011.

86. Coughlin ME, Gibbins S, Hoath SB. Core measures for developmentally supportive care in neonatal intensive care units: theory, precedence and practice. J Adv Nurs. 2009;65(10):2239–48.

87. Staniszewska S, Brett J, Redshaw M, Hamilton K, Newburn M, Jones N, et al. The POPPY study: developing a model of family-centred care for neonatal units. Worldviews Evid Based Nurs. 2012;2012:243–55. https://doi.org/10.1111/j.1741-6787.2012.00253.x.

88. Altimier L, Phillips R. The neonatal integrative developmental care model: advanced clinical applications of the seven core measures for neuroprotective family-centered developmental care. Newborn Infant Nurs Rev. 2016;16(4):230–44. https://doi.org/10.1053/j.nainr.2016.09.030.

89. Roué JM, Kuhn P, Lopez Maestro M, Maastrup RA, Mitanchez D, Westrup B, et al. Eight principles for patient-centred and family-centred care for newborns in the neonatal intensive care unit. Arch Dis Child Fetal Neonat Ed. 2017;102(4):F364–8. https://doi.org/10.1136/archdischild-2016-312180.

90. Dai K, Fan X, Shi H, Xiong X, Ding L, Yu Y, et al. Application of family-centered empowerment model in primary caregivers of premature infants: a quasi-experimental study. Front Pediatr. 2023;11:1137188. https://doi.org/10.3389/fped.2023.1137188.

91. British Association of Perinatal Medicine (BAPM). Family integrated care a framework for practice. London: BAPM; 2021. https://www.bapm.org/resources/ficare-framework-for-practice. Accessed 12 August 2024

92. Pittiruti M, Van Boxtel T, Scoppettuolo G, Carr P, Konstantinou E, Ortiz Miluy G, et al. European recommendations on the proper indication and use of peripheral venous access devices (the ERPIUP consensus): a WoCoVA project. J Vasc Access. 2023;24(1):165–82. https://doi.org/10.1177/11297298211023274.

93. Pittiruti M, Crocoli A, Zanaboni C, Annetta MG, Bevilacqua M, Biasucci DG, et al. The pediatric DAV-expert algorithm: a GAVeCeLT/GAVePed consensus for the choice of the most appropriate venous access device in children. J Vasc Access. 2024;10:11297298241256999. https://doi.org/10.1177/11297298241256999.

94. Fernández-Fernández I, Castro-Sánchez E, Blanco-Mavillard I. Determinants of the optimal selection of vascular access devices: a systematic review underpinned by the COM-B behavioural model. J Adv Nurs. 2024; https://doi.org/10.1111/jan.16202.

95. Krein SL, Kuhn L, Ratz D, Chopra V. Use of designated nurse PICC teams and CLABSI prevention practices among U.S. hospitals: a survey-based study. J Patient Saf. 2019;15(4):293–5. https://doi.org/10.1097/PTS.0000000000000246.

96. Bayoumi MAA, Van Rens MFP, Chandra P, Francia ALV, D'Souza S, George M, et al. Effect of implementing an epicutaneo-caval catheter team in neonatal intensive care unit. J Vasc Access. 2021;22(2):243–53. https://doi.org/10.1177/1129729820928182.

97. van Rens MFPT, Hugill K, Gaffari MAK, Francia AV, Ramkumar T, Garcia KLP, et al. Outcomes of establishing a neonatal peripheral vascular access team. Arch Dis Child Fetal Neonat Ed. 2021;108(1):F88–9. https://doi.org/10.1136/fetalneonatal-2021-322764.

98. The National Infusion and Vascular Access Society (NIVAS). The Benefits of a nursing led vascular access service team: a white paper to outline a standardised structure and approach for the NHS to deliver vascular access services in every hospital, June 2022. https://nivas.org.uk/contentimages/main/NIVAS-White-paper-for-standardisation-of-vascular-access-teams-within-the-NHS_FINAL-27.06.22.pdf. Accessed 12 August 2024.

99. Ullman AJ, Bernstein SJ, Brown E, Aiyagari R, Doellman D, Faustino EVS, et al. The Michigan appropriateness guide for intravenous catheters in pediatrics: miniMAGIC. Pediatrics. 2020;145(Suppl 3):S269–84. https://doi.org/10.1542/peds.2019-3474I.

100. Osmond E, Williams N. Fifteen-minute consultation: decision-making pathway for neonatal vascular access. Arch Dis Child Educ Pract Ed. 2022;107(4):242–5. https://doi.org/10.1136/archdischild-2020-320136.

101. van Rens MFPT, Bayoumi MA, van de Hoogen A, Francia ALV, Cabanillas IJ, van Loon FHJ, et al. The ABBA project (assess better before access): a retrospective, cross-sectional study of neonatal intravascular device outcomes. Front Pediatr. 2022;10:10.980725. https://doi.org/10.3389/fped.2022.980725.

102. Barone G, D'Andrea V, Ancora G, Cresi F, Maggio L, Capasso A, et al. The neonatal DAV-expert algorithm: a GAVeCeLT/GAVePed consensus for the choice of the most appropriate venous access in newborns. Eur J Pediatr. 2023;182(8):3385–95. https://doi.org/10.1007/s00431-023-04984-4.

103. Centers for Disease Control and Prevention (CDC). Background information: catheter types from the guidelines for the prevention of intravascular catheter-related infections, 2011. https://www.cdc.gov/infection-control/hcp/intravascular-catheter-related-infection/table-1-catheter-types.html. Accessed 12 August 2024

104. van Rens M, van der Lee R, Spencer TR, van Boxtel T, Barone G, Crocoli A, et al. The NAVIGATE project: a GloVANet–WoCoVA position statement on the nomenclature for vascular access devices. J Vasc Access. 2024; https://doi.org/10.1177/11297298241291248.

Optimising Neonatal Vascular Access

Technology in Vascular Access

3

Chapter Learning Objectives

Upon completing this chapter, readers will be able to:

- Critically evaluate the value and limitations of health technology aids in vascular access.
  - In relation to choosing the optimal: vascular access route, blood vessel health, vascular device insertion, infusion control, and monitoring to detect complications.
- Advocate for evidence-based protocol driven approaches when using advanced technologies.
  - In relation to aiding vascular health assessment, device insertion, ensuring infusion safety, and insertion site monitoring.
- Promote the integration of health technology aids into practice to improve the success, safety, and overall outcomes of neonatal vascular access.
- Critically reflect on the challenges associated with using and embedding health technologies into everyday neonatal vascular access practice.

3.1 Introduction

The application of existing and newly discovered scientific knowledge in novel ways to solve practical problems defines technology. The modern world cannot function without technology in all its guises, and this includes healthcare. Ideas about technology and how it can be categorised are constantly evolving. One way is to categorise technology into broad types or family groupings. However, each of these groupings can be confusingly, inconsistently, and interchangeably defined. In relation to vascular access, important groupings include aeronautical (or space) technology, material science technology, biotechnology, biomedical engineering, information and computer technology, pharmaceutical science technology, and

© The Author(s), under exclusive license to Springer Nature
Switzerland AG 2024
M. R. van Rens, K. Hugill, *Vascular Access in Neonatal Nursing Practice:
A Neuroprotective Approach*, https://doi.org/10.1007/978-3-031-81602-4_3

applied educational technologies such as augmented/virtual reality. When referring to the application of technology, key terms include 'low', 'high', 'intermediate', though again most of these terms are variously defined and applied.

Health technology can change healthcare provider and patient behaviours but is primarily focused on solving the problems of preventative healthcare, targeted diagnosis of health problems, delivering better performing treatments, ensuring patient safety, and preventing complications. Health economics, sustainability, and being environmentally less damaging are also key foci.

3.1.1 Impacts of Technology

Technology takes many forms and sometimes its effects cannot be entirely predicted. One example: Sir Tim Berners-Lee working at the European Organization for Nuclear Research, better known as CERN, developed in 1989 computer code to share information automatically between scientists. This innovation was made available to other scientific research institutions in 1991 and later in 1993 to the public, patent and royalty free. The computer code is better known today as the 'World Wide Web' or in its abbreviated form 'WWW' [1].

In healthcare, an example of technology impacting beyond its intended use is the following account. Godfrey N Howfield and Allan M Cormack, an engineer and a physicist were initially met with scepticism and dismissed as eccentrics by the medical establishment for their groundbreaking work in clinical imaging [2, 3]. Together they are credited with developing the first commercially available computer-assisted tomography, better known by the abbreviated 'CT scanner'. A development so significant and now seen as a lynchpin of health diagnostics that they were jointly awarded the 1979 Nobel Prize in Physiology or Medicine [3].

When plastic single use items became readily available [4], this influenced healthcare providers practices around infusion therapy in significant ways and contributed to the ubiquity of vascular access now seen. In neonatology following a great deal of research and development, synthetic surfactant became a viable treatment for newborn respiratory distress syndrome (NRDS) [5–7]. Now surfactant administration is incorporated into routine use in neonatal intensive care units (NICUs) across the world. This development has led to a near elimination of a leading cause of premature infant death and contributed to the long-term survival of extremely preterm and smaller infants.

At the time of their initial dissemination, the impacts of these examples of technological innovation on everyday life and health care were underappreciated. Together they represent a group known as 'disruptive' or 'transformative' technologies. This is a category of technology so named as its introduction overturns preexisting business models, ways of doing things, or how people see the world and its possibilities. Whilst many technological innovations and their promoters claim to be disruptive or transformative, the reality is that few are truly that momentous (Text Box 3.1).

Text Box 3.1 Practice Point: Being Pragmatic About Health Technology
Incorporating incremental advances of existing technologies or evaluating the potential utility of applying technologies from other family groupings could be beneficial for patient outcomes.

- But every innovation needs considered, contextual evaluation before its adoption to avoid unintended adverse effects.

Remaining cognizant of emerging wider social and technological synergies such as artificial intelligence (AI), quantum computing, and augmented (AR)/virtual (VR) reality tools, e.g., could lead to new opportunities for developing vascular access practices.

3.2   Technological Approaches to Vascular Access Device Design and Manufacture

3.2.1   Catheter Design and Material

Though seldom consciously factored into decision-making, catheter material and design can impact the likelihood of device-related complications and unplanned removal [8–11]. It is therefore essential to take into consideration the properties and characteristics of different device materials and design options to ensure that informed choices are tailored to individual patient, clinical, and therapeutic needs. Biocompatibility, non-toxicity, and chemical inertness are essential prerequisites of all vascular access devices and catheters. Commonly used PVAD and CVAD device materials include polyurethane (PUR), polytetrafluoroethylene (PTFE), fluoroethylene polypropylene (FEP), and silicone. Each material offers distinct advantages and disadvantages that make them more or less suitable for specific clinical scenarios.

3.2.1.1 Polyether Block Amide (PEBA)
This material is less commonly used in neonatal settings due to its inherent stiffness and high resistance to collapse which could prove problematic in small blood vessels. However, when these attributes are desired such as undampened pressure waveforms or longer catheter lengths are required (e.g., n-LPC or arterial catheters), the material has a role whereby overly compliant catheter materials like silicone or PUR would be less desirable [12].

3.2.1.2 Silicone
Silicone catheters typically have a soft and smooth inner and outer surface; these characteristics are reported to have thromboresistant properties, enhance patient comfort during long-term use, and reduce the risk of vessel trauma and mechanical

irritation. However, n-PICC/ECCs made from silicone are thought to underperform when compared to PUR catheters and have fallen out of favour in practice [13].

3.2.1.3 Polytetrafluoroethylene (PTFE)

PTFE is a synthetic fluoropolymer marketed under the brand name Teflon™. This chemical has an exceptionally low coefficient of friction, and this combined with its inherent kink resistance can reduce resistance during insertion. Additionally, PTFE exhibits thromboresistant properties, leading to a reduced tendency to promote blood clot formation on its surface. However, its relative rigidity compared to other materials is thought to be a cause of the higher incidence of mechanical phlebitis reported from devices made from PTFE [14].

3.2.1.4 Fluorinated Ethylene Polypropylene (FEP)

It is a newer formulation with properties very close to those exhibited by PTFE but without some of the limitations of PTFE. It is notably softer and less stiff than PTFE. FEP formulations are marketed under a variety of commercial brand names depending on the formula owners, including Teflon™ FEP, Neoflon™ FEP, and Dyneon™/3M™ FEP. In its various proprietary formulations, it can be found in Jelco® (Smiths Medical) and Clip®Neosafe I.V. (Greiner Bio-One) PVADs.

3.2.1.5 Polyurethane (PUR)

PUR is best considered as a generic term for a class of chemically related polymers that can be modified during manufacture to show desirable properties. PUR can be chemically modified to be transparent or radiopaque, thermoplastic, flexible, and kink-resistant. In general, PUR exhibits properties that make it well-suited for various medical applications, including vascular access devices.

In vascular access flexibility can greatly enable ease of insertion and reduce the risk of vessel damage during placement, whilst kink resistance can help maintain stable fluid flow and reduce the risk of catheter occlusion. However, over time (in use or storage), PUR can become less pliable which may increase the risk of vessel irritation or perforation. This can make PUR less suitable for devices intended for prolonged (years) use without thought given to their periodic replacement.

Vialon™ is a proprietary formulation of PUR owned by the medical product manufacturer Becton Dickinson and Company (BD). It is incorporated into many of their vascular access devices. The material is bio-reactive and softens after insertion at body temperatures by up to 70%. This feature is thought to account for the reduced risk of mechanical phlebitis reported in numerous studies [15, 16].

Meta-analysis of pooled data from 7 studies (n = 3724 adult participants, 4281 PVADs) found that devices made from Vialon (with integrated or closed systems, or wings) compared to designs made from Teflon (that were not integrated, or without wings) performed better [17]. However, these results should be interpreted with caution. Five studies had less than 400 participants each and the individual studies showed considerable heterogenicity and variability in outcome measures, making generalisations to other settings and patient populations impractical.

The acceptability of any treatment intervention affects patient satisfaction and treatment outcomes. Vascular access procedures are a cause of pain and anxiety for infants and parents. This can affect infant behaviour and parents' ability to provide comfort for their infant during the procedure. Offering reassurance, clear explanations, and taking measures to reduce pain experiences can be helpful and improve infant and parent experience. One small study ($n = 208$) using a randomised trial design [18] investigated the effects on pain intensity scores from using PVADs made from two common materials, Teflon and Vialon. In this study, the reported pain intensity scores were similar between the two groups, suggesting that PVAD material has little effect on patient pain experience at the time of insertion. However, analysis of secondary outcomes established that PVADs made from Vialon were associated with longer dwell times and less phlebitis (16.3% versus 53.8% for Teflon) [18]. Phlebitis is painful and leads to unplanned PVAD removal and possible reinsertion. Designs incorporating Vialon could result in lower overall vascular access associated pain due to less phlebitis and fewer repeated insertions.

PUR in various proprietary formulations is present in a range of neonatal PVADs and central line catheters, including SuperCath® (ICU Medical), Introcan Safety® (Braun), Versatus® range (Terumo), the BD Neoflon™ (Becton Dickinson), and the Vygon range of n-PICC/ECCs. Newer innovative developments in vascular access devices involve combining different catheter materials. These hybrid devices aim to offer enhanced performance and improved patient outcomes. The results of clinical evaluations when available will be most welcome (Text Box 3.2).

Text Box 3.2 Practice Point: Selecting the Best Vascular Access Device
There is no single correct choice of vascular access device.

- Typically, however, using the smallest size catheter and the fewest number of lumens suitable for the intended therapy can be a helpful pointer.

  Vascular access device materials have unique characteristics that make them suitable for specific clinical situations and less suitable for others.
  Selection of the most appropriate catheter material is contextual and informed by patient and therapy-specific factors.

3.2.2   Advanced Design Features

Advanced design features such as optional wings, visual confirmation of lumen entry, access ports, needlestick injury prevention, and the like play an important role in ensuring the safety of healthcare providers and patients and the efficacy of vascular access procedures. Other advanced features include in-line infusion filters, values (of various design), antiseptic barrier caps, and infusion regulating pumps (which are considered in Chaps. 4 and 5.

3.2.2.1 Infusion Filters and Valves

Infusion filters and valves as used in vascular access devices are available in a variety of patented and trademarked designs and marketing names. Each device purportedly has distinct advantages over its competitors' products. Despite the many valve options available, several generic design principles are evident. These include 'backcheck values' (also known as anti-syphon or one-way), 'slit valves' (also known as split septum or self-sealing), and 'flow controlling valves (also known as flow control or rate control). The intent of all these designs is to regulate fluid flow direction and perform as a barrier. This can be to:

- Maintain unidirectional flow
- Prevent retrograde flow
- Prevent microbial contamination
- Prevent air emboli and microplastics entering infusions
- Reduce needlestick injury risk
- Enable or prevent fluid and blood sampling
- Minimise blood loss during access
- Customise and ensure consistent precise flow rates

with the intent to improve patient and user safety and prolong catheter use.

In-line infusion filters are considered to be essential features of most infusion circuits. They are designed to remove particulate matter (including suspended plastics and glass particles), air from the infusion circuit, bacterial endotoxins, or lipid aggregates [19].

A Cochrane review in 2015 [20] of four randomised or quasi-randomised studies failed to endorse their routine use in neonatal settings, citing a lack of robust high-quality evidence. More recent work has also failed to arrive at a definite consensus and fully endorse the use of in-line filtration devices to prevent phlebitis or reduce exposure to biologically 'inert' substances [21]. This is in part due to a lack of contemporary clinical studies. However, the use of in-line filtration for neonates receiving parenteral nutrition was concluded to be likely beneficial in reducing systemic inflammatory complications and therefore tentatively endorsed [21].

3.2.2.2 Antiseptic Barrier Caps

Accessing and manipulating vascular catheters to change infusions or administer bolus injections is a known risk for complications, particularly infection [22]. The technique of 'Scrub-the-Hub' used before accessing vascular lines is widely considered to be an essential component of good ANTT® practice (e.g., [23–26]) and is firmly established in many NICUs.

Antiseptic barrier caps, sometimes referred to as port protectors containing 70% isopropyl alcohol or chlorhexidine solutions are marketed under several trademark protected names. These devices address a common problem in practice, needleless catheter hub, and connector contamination. A situation further exacerbated if there is poor compliance with hub disinfection procedures before access. This presents a potential intraluminal route for infection to enter the bloodstream. Gillis and colleagues [27] in a systematic review and meta-analysis of 16/15 studies examined the use of antiseptic barrier caps with peripheral inserted central lines (PICC) on the incidence of central line-associated bloodstream infection (CLABSI). They concluded that whilst most studies had methodological weaknesses and that more robust data is needed, antiseptic barrier caps were safe, easy to use, readily acceptable to staff and patients, and a cost-effective addition to CLABSI prevention strategies [27]. However, although the sample size included children, all were post-neonatal in age, and none of the research settings was an NICU, making the transferability of these findings to this patient group uncertain.

Even at term-corrected ages, infants born preterm still exhibit poorer skin integrity [28]. This suggests that epidermal barrier maturation is dependent on developmental processes influenced by gestational age and the time from birth. In addition, newborn skin has peculiar and non-linear absorption characteristics to topically applied medications and chemicals [29]. An unpredictable situation could prove hazardous when infant skin is exposed to topically applied chemicals. Several in vitro bench studies have raised concerns about risks and unintended consequences from using alcohol containing antiseptic barrier caps with neonatal patients [30, 31]. This concern is due to the ingress of alcohol into the catheter (and patient bloodstream), leading to a risk of alcohol toxicity, a rare but documented risk in preterm infants [32–35].

Boissière et al. [32] in a bench study examined the impact of using different combinations of alcohol disinfection caps alone and in combination with a variety of needleless connectors manufactured by different companies. No cap had zero leakage. The likelihood of leakage was time dependent, and the amount was related to the loading volume of alcohol in the individual cap, which varied between devices. Caps used in combination with the same manufacturer's needleless connectors tended to have less leakage. Suggesting that using matched devices might reduce risks. However, whilst in testing, alcohol leaks into the catheter, and consequently, the patients' bloodstream was generally negligible, the risk was never zero. Consequently, the authors urge caution when using alcohol disinfection caps with paediatric and neonatal patients.

Results from research indicate that antiseptic barrier caps provide additional protection from intraluminal contamination and possibly bloodstream infection [27]. However, in NICUs, concern about the potential for inadvertence exposure of infants to alcohol toxicity is unresolved. In the absence of consensus about the safety of antiseptic barrier caps, then caution in their use to avoid leakage and vigilance for toxicity is essential. Examining published studies demonstrate that consensus about the use of antiseptic barrier caps with neonatal aged patients is lacking. It seems likely that the optimal design for these devices is not yet achieved, and further innovations and refinements can be expected. Further research is needed to ascertain the safety and effectiveness of using these devices to prevent hub and intraluminal contamination across the range of gestational ages seen in NICU patients.

In-line filtration devices and antiseptic caps have theoretical advantages in improving patient well-being and safety. However, their utility in NICU settings is not fully established and their use is not risk free (Text Box 3.3).

Text Box 3.3 Practice Point: Using Advanced Infusion Aids in the NICU
The evidence supporting the use of in-line filtration devices in neonatal vascular access practice and the safety of antiseptic barrier caps is inconclusive and underdeveloped, excluding the use of in-line filters for parenteral nutrition.

Careful consideration of the supporting evidence-base balanced with an understanding of local contexts and patient risk factors is required for the safe, efficient, and economic use of these important devices.

3.3 Technological Approaches for Ensuring Safe Insertion of Vascular Access Devices

3.3.1 Aiding Better PVAD Insertion

When deciding upon which blood vessel to use for a PVAD, it is essential to avoid using blood vessels reserved for n-PICC/ECC insertion (such as the long saphenous veins or those in the antecubital fossa) or those previously damaged by needlestick. Neonates are prone to developing difficult venous access. Protocol-led systematic assessment of vessel health and suitability (e.g., rapid superficial vein assessment, RaSuVA) is essential to maximise patient safety and ensure insertion success [36, 37]. The results of pre-procedural assessments should be incorporated into vascular access planning and can also contribute to measures to rationalise vein use and preserve blood vessels, their use is commended.

3.3.1.1 Vein Visualisation
When superficial blood vessels are difficult to visualise or palpate, there are several technologies that can help including near-infrared and transillumination devices. Near-infrared spectroscopy (NIRS) is used to non-invasively measure regional tissue oxygenation and provide early notification of tissue perfusion issues in surgery and critical illness (e.g., [38, 39]). One development of this technology is now available to assist in the visualisation of peripheral venous blood vessels (near-infrared (NIR) illumination) [40]. These devices project light of various near-infrared wavelengths onto the skin surface, enabling the user to see a dynamic real-time image of the superficial vasculature and surrounding tissues. Advocates propose that NIR devices designed for detecting veins can reveal wider selection of veins for vascular access than using other methods, detect the presence of valves in veins, improve first-attempt success rates, and reduce the number of attempts before successful insertion of PVADs. However, research evidence is conflicted on the relative merits of the different commercial products and technologies.

Rothbart and colleagues [41] examined the use of one device, the AccuVein® AV300 vein viewer (AccuVein®, LLC, 40 Goose hill Rd., Cold Spring Harbour, NY, USA). In their study, presurgical patients aged between 0 and 17 years ($n = 238$) had vascular access device inserted into veins identified by the NIR vein viewer. Sadly, first-attempt success rates fell from 73% to 45% when using the device only. This finding replicates that from an earlier unrelated study [42]. Explanations for this result were attributed to a lack of targeted training, unfamiliarity with the technique and equipment, limited experience affecting dexterity in use (an assistant held device), and skill in interpretation of the image and depth perception. Only 31 participants were between 0 and 3 months of age, making it difficult to apply these findings to neonatal settings.

A randomised controlled trial involving 115 neonates reported that the vein viewer device performed better on more advanced gestational age infants than those of a younger and presumably smaller gestational age [43]. In contrast, another NICU-based study [44] reported that with infants >2.5 kg, there was no difference in first-attempt success rates between using standard approaches for vein visualisation (56.1%) and NIR (60.6%) methods, except amongst less experienced nurses (1 year NICU working). Interestingly, this subgroup of nurses achieved better first-attempt success rates, moving from a 23.1% first-attempt success rate to 72.7%; a figure that exceeds the unit average [44]. This finding is surprising and warrants further investigation to ascertain reasons for this. Speculatively, it could reflect differences in educational preparation for working in an NICU, age-related visual changes, or differences in the acceptance to using technology, amongst other explanations.

Clinician-modified transillumination light sources have been used in the past to aid diagnosis of pneumothorax and help to identify veins in patients with difficult vascular access. However, these early devices were associated with significant risks of causing thermal burns if left in contact with the skin for too long. Newer and safer bespoke designs suitable for use with neonates are now available, some using LED technology. Transillumination-based vein visualisation aids (e.g., Veinlite Neo® transillumination device—Translite LLC, Sugar Land, TX, USA, and Wee Sight®—Respironics Inc., Koninklijke Philips N.V., Amsterdam, The Netherlands) use LED generated light to penetrate tissues and create an image of the anatomy. This allows healthcare providers to see blood vessels. These devices have significant cost benefits over NIR vein viewing devices, being considerably less expensive. There is some evidence from small studies that using LED-based transillumination devices can help to improve first-attempt success rates amongst infants and small children less than 2 years old from 49% to 73% [45]. However, there are few studies that have sought to compare NIR and transillumination in neonatal populations.

One study used a randomised trial design to compare IRS, transillumination, or standards care in a group of preterm infants ($n = 90$). Both IRS and transillumination use led to improved first-attempt success rates compared to standard care, and IRS use improved dwell time. However, transillumination was associated with statistically more patient handling time and higher patient pain scores than either IRS or standard care [46]. The findings are interesting and could be used to guide purchasing decisions and guideline development (Text Box 3.4).

Text Box 3.4 Practice Point: Visualising Difficult to See Veins
Both NIR light projection, transillumination, and ultrasound based vein visualisation technologies have the potential to offer valuable contributions and aid healthcare providers locate and assess the suitability of blood vessels for vascular access procedures.

3.3.2   Aiding Better CVAD Insertion

CVADs in neonates include the familiar UVC, n-PICC/ECC, and for many nurses working outside of specialist units, until quite recently, the less usually encountered CICC, FICC, and tunnelled devices. Traditional radiography, using a portable X-ray machine can confirm CVAD tip position by interpreting its location relative to anatomical markers. However, there are limitations to this approach. X-rays involve exposure to ionising radiation, are invariably not in 'real-time', and can be open to miss interpretation due to rotated or lordotic images. Newer applications of ultrasound and ECG technology are establishing themselves as the standard for confirmation of catheter tip, and their use has additional benefits.

3.3.2.1 Ultrasound

Ultrasound uses soundwaves of varying frequencies emitted and reflected through a transducer to image soft tissues, including blood vessels and surrounding tissues. Software and transducer refinements can detect blood flow based on shifts in frequency using the Doppler effect. First used in a department-based diagnostic capacity, ultrasound machines are now available for use at the bedside, the so-called point-of-care ultrasound (POCUS). POCUS is now widely used for bedside diagnosis and to support invasive clinical procedures in critical care settings, including NICUs [47].

In vascular access, ultrasound is considered a versatile tool allowing healthcare providers to visualise the peripheral and deep vasculature in detail [48, 49]. During these ultrasound-led assessments, it is possible to identify and rule out stenosed, thrombotic, anatomically abnormal blood vessels [50–52]. In contrast to other vein visualisation technologies, ultrasound can determine variations in lumen calibre, vessel depth, anatomical shape, and the proximity of additional tissues (nerves, arteries, etc.) that might affect catheter insertion.

Standardised protocols can be used to evaluate the suitability of blood vessels for vascular access. Currently, protocols include the Rapid Central Vein Assessment (RaCeVA) [50], the Rapid Femoral Vein Assessment (RaFeVA) [51], and the Rapid Assessment of Vascular Exit Site and Tunnelling Options (RAVESTO) [52]. In essence, RaCeVA bilaterally evaluates the four central veins that could feasibly be accessed in neonates (internal and external jugular, subclavian, and brachiocephalic veins). RaFeVA follows a similar schematic but focuses upon the blood vessels of the lower limbs, whilst the RAVESTO protocol seeks to appraise the optimal exit site for subcutaneously tunnelled CICC and FICCs.

The major benefit of using POCUS is to guide catheter insertion and tip navigation (tunnelled and non-tunnelled) in real-time using dynamic information to confirm correct placement [53–55]. There are reports of using ultrasound to redirect misdirected catheters during insertion [56]. Doing this will avoid having to remove the catheter, saving time and money, ensuring a prompt start to therapy, reducing pain and discomfort and promoting a better patient experience, and possibly reducing parental anxiety. This technology when used by experienced operators can improve insertion success rates, ensure correct catheter tip location, and help to avoid complications like catheter misplacement or vessel wall perforation. However, effective use requires the availability of appropriate equipment suitable for use with neonate, robust evidence-based guidelines, structured protocols, and training and skill in use [48, 57–59].

3.3.2.2 Intracavity Electrocardiogram

Intracavity electrocardiogram (IC-ECG) guided insertion techniques help determine the correct placement of the CVAD tip by using changes in the ECG signal. Specifically, the P wave changes in a predictable and distinctive way as the catheter tip enters superior vena cava, cavoatrial junction, and right atrium [60]. The technique is suitable for use with neonates, so long as the P wave is present in the ECG trace [61].

Studies of the effectiveness of IC-ECG are positive. One study compared IC-ECG and conventional X-radiography. In this study, IC-ECG was more successful in achieving optimal catheter tip placement and was associated with fewer catheter-related complications (3.75% versus 23.75%) [62]. Another small (n = 161) study involving neonates [63] and a nurse-led n-PICC/ECC insertion team using similar evaluation criteria to the previous study reported largely comparable results. This study reported statistically significant findings for better initial optimal placement of catheter tip (93.59%—IC-ECG versus 73.49%—conventional) and fewer overall catheter-related complications (3.84%—IC-ECG versus 14.46%—conventional). Subgroup analysis of individual complications did not provide statistically significant findings [63]. It seems probably that combining IC-ECG guidance with ultrasound imaging might further enhance procedural success and safety [64] (Text Box 3.5).

Text Box 3.5 Practice Point: POCUS and ECG-Guided Vascular Access in Neonates

The integration of POCUS and IC-ECG-guided technologies into neonatal central vascular access has led to an increased variety of vascular access options in this patient group, more precise catheter placement, and reduced risk of insertion-related complications.

POCUS requires a dedicated period of learning engagement for users to become competent. In contrast, IC-ECG is a safe, reliable, and comparatively easy technique to learn and use.

3.3.3 Aiding Better Securement of PVADs and CVADs

Historically neonatal vascular access devices were secured with a variety of tapes (often non-sterile), wraps, gauze dressings, and sutures [65]. This situation inevitably led to inadequate securement and insertion site protection. Consequently, this resulted in problems with catheter movement and dislodgment, mechanical phlebitis, fluid infiltration, medical adhesive related skin injury (MARSI), and extraluminal infection. Such approaches are no longer considered acceptable and have been largely abandoned.

Newer evidence-based ideas about how best to secure catheters and dress insertion sites to improve device stability and reduce infection risk have been widely studied and recommended for practice [25, 66–71]. This should reduce unexplained practice variation.

Effective securement of PVAD and CVADs ensures their proper performance and reduces complications. Engineered solutions including adherent skin surface and sutureless subcutaneously anchored devices are popular choices [25, 65–68, 70, 71], though securement to compromised neonatal skin remains challenging. For example, the Clik-FIX® (Braun) used in combination with a PUR transparent and semipermeable dressing or combined securement and dressing kits. Of which the 3M-Tegaderm advanced securement dressing (Solventum) is an example. Some dressing designs are available with embedded chlorhexidine gel or pads to help prevent infection. A recent National Institute for Health and Care Excellence (NICE) Medical technology innovation briefing concluded that chlorhexidine pads and gel dressing formulations are generally not suitable for children below 2 months of age [72]. For neonates, additional concerns about hypersensitivity and skin necrosis are evident, and consequently, their use is not recommended [72]. One novel technological innovation that has established a role in vascular device securement is tissue adhesive.

3.3.3.1 Medical Grade Cyanoacrylate Tissue Adhesive

Cyanoacrylate-based adhesives are invariably clear colourless liquids with a strong irritant odour and form strong bonds between in contact surfaces due to polymerisation (curing) when exposed to moisture. Different chemical formulations can be engineered to have unique adherence characteristics, breaking strengths, and flexibility. These adhesives have many applications in industrial and domestic settings.

Medical grade cyanoacrylate adhesives are made from intermediate chain butyl cyanoacrylate, long chain octyl cyanoacrylate, or sometimes a combination of both compounds (octyl-butyl-cyanoacrylate). These formulations are biocompatible and avoid the toxicities associated with other consumer and industrial cyanoacrylate formulations [73]. Medical quality formulations of cyanoacrylate have a proven safety record and naturally lose their adherence over a period of around 5–7 days as the skin naturally regenerates. However, this can necessitate reapplication to ensure continued adhesion, though overapplication should be avoided [74]. Cyanoacrylate-based tissue adhesives have established a role in traumatic and surgical wound closure as an alternative to sutures and as an aid for securing vascular catheters and lines [25].

One preparation made from a mixture of 2-octyl cyanoacrylate and n-butyl-2-cyanoacrylate is approved for use in vascular access in the USA, UK, and Europe. This compound is marked as SecurePortIV® (H.B. Fuller Medical Adhesive Technologies, Saint Paul MN USA). It is currently the only product licensed for all vascular access devices and for use with all patient age groups [74]. In addition to providing securement and improved dressing integrity, application of the adhesive also seals the catheter exit site at the skin surface, provides haemostasis, and immobilises skin flora; this might mitigate infection risks associated with skin breaking procedures [75–80].

In neonatal, research into adhesive use for catheter securement has been done for CVADs (e.g., [76, 77]) and PVADs [78]. Van Rens et al. [77] studied using cyanoacrylate for n-PICC/ECC securement following 1842 successful insertions (867 using additional tissue adhesive and 975 using standard dressing securement alone). The addition of cyanoacrylate for catheter securement resulted in fewer cases of therapy failure compared to standard care. However, randomised controlled trials comparing different adhesive formulations used alone or in combination with other securement devices have yet to be conducted [79]. One large neonatal retrospective study ($n = 8330$ PVADs) compared transparent dressing securement with the same dressing but with adjunct use of tissue adhesive [78]. Results concerning the two interventions suggested unplanned early removal, device-related phlebitis were statistically significant in favour of using tissue adhesive [78]. If early removal is necessary, say due to therapy completion or unplanned removal, then using a gentle rolling motion can achieve sufficient debonding to enable catheter removal. It is not necessary to removal all the adhesive residue unless clinically indicated [81] (Text Box 3.6).

Text Box 3.6 Practice Point: Cyanoacrylate Tissue Adhesive for PVAD and CVAD Securement in Neonates

Cyanoacrylate tissue adhesive aids catheter securement and provides haemostasis and an additional layer of protection against infection by restricting extraluminal contamination from bacterial migration.

Cyanoacrylate tissue adhesive is recommended as the standard of care for vascular access device securement and as an adjunct for dressing fixation.

In neonates, the adhesives are safe and easy to apply and they naturally separate over time as the epidermis exfoliates. Early removal, if required can be achieved by using a gentle rolling motion, though it is generally best to wait for natural separation.

3.4   Technological Aids Ensuring Safe Infusion

Despite improvements in prevention, diagnosis and treatment infiltration and extravasation injuries in infants in NICU continue to present serious concerns for healthcare providers. Several technologies can be applied to reduce these risks including infusion pump control and pressure monitoring (explored in Chap. 5), human-led observational tools, and sensing technologies for earlier notification of complications.

3.4.1   Sensing Technologies

Research into sensing technologies for the detection of fluid infiltration and extravasation from blood vessel during infusion are becoming more prevalent in the literature. Approaches for the detection of peripheral fluid infusion infiltration are based on several different engineering technologies (Fig. 3.1) [82]. Whilst some of these are still at the laboratory bench stage or used in biomedical research, some have become commercially available. These devices provide real-time information and continuous monitoring of the insertion site and can be used to complement existing visual and tactile inspections to improve early notification of PIVIE events.

Many of the technologies aimed at detecting infiltration are still under research, but some such as ultrasound and optical sensing have been commercialised for clinically useful application [82]. Ensuring sensitivity and specificity in detecting the very small volume changes such as seen with preterm infant infiltration/extravasation events are challenging. One device is reported as capable of detecting small volume changes in superficial veins with clinically useful levels of sensitivity and

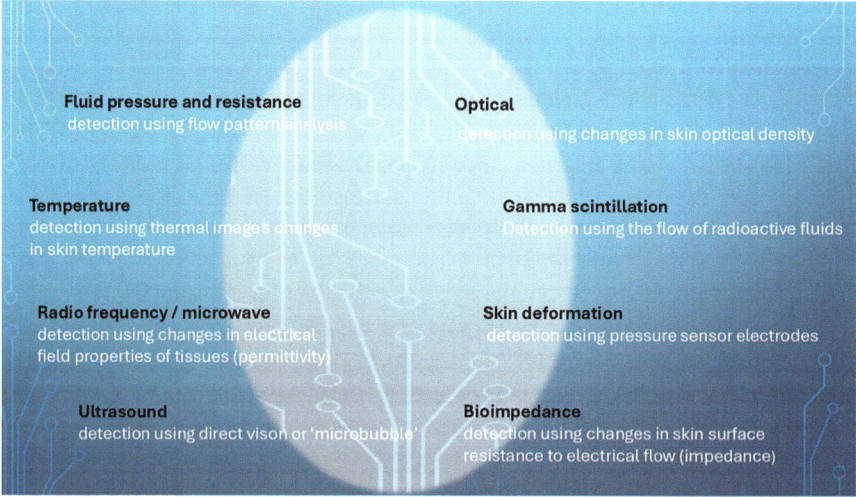

Fig. 3.1 Sensing technologies for PIVIE detection

specificity. This device, approved in the USA, UK, and Europe for use in neonatal populations uses optical sensor technology, the ivWatch (ivWatch LLC, Newport News, VA. USA).

This system uses a combined NIR and visible light LED light source and sensor. The sensor is located on the skin surface near to the height of the PVAD tip and on the left or right of the tip but not immediately above it. The device allows continuous site monitoring. An interpretive software algorithm is used to detect changes in the optical properties of the monitored site and alert healthcare providers to check the insertion site for a possible infiltration event [83–85]. A small number of studies in paediatric and neonatal critical care settings have been done or proposed (e.g., [86–90]). One pilot study in a Middle Eastern country's NICU continuously monitored the infusion of a small number of vesicant infusions [88]. The authors found the device detected 14 out of 15 PIVIE events confirmed by TLC inspection (sensitivity 93.3%). All the 14 PIVIEs detected were notified earlier than the time detected by nurses. D'Andrea et al. [89] piloting the device with a preterm infant study group reported a sensitivity of 88.9% and a specificity of 84.4%, noting notification occurred 6 h before staff detected a PIVIE. A European study with a low baseline incidence of PIVIE (3.25%) reported similar conclusions [90], detecting 113 PIVIEs from 3476 PVADs (100% sensitivity) with all events detected (100% sensitivity), again before healthcare provider confirmation (Text Box 3.7).

Text Box 3.7 Practice Point: Detecting PIVIE Using Optical Sensor Technology
Optical sensor technologies for the detection of peripheral vascular infiltration are safe and simple to use and exhibit high levels of sensitivity and specificity when used with neonatal patients.

Advanced optical sensor technology can be readily integrated with existing observational tools such as TLC. Doing this adds an additional layer of observation ensuring earlier detection and reduced severity of PIVIE events. This can enhance patient safety, elevate care experiences, and the overall quality of care for neonates requiring peripheral vascular access.

3.5   Technology and Its Impacts on NICU Parents

NICUs can be characterised by the presence of advanced healthcare technology, a high work pace and critical decision-making [91]. Whilst people will react individually, early NICU experience can affect subsequent parental behaviours, prolong feelings of distress, and affect levels of satisfaction. Nonetheless, the technology of the NICU environment is consistently reported to be intimidating for parents during what is an emotionally upsetting and disorienting time in their lives (e.g., [92–97]). In contrast, one ethnographic study of parents (fathers) in NICU observed that some participants vigilantly watched the monitoring technology and how out of parameter alarms were acted upon. Participants stated they found the presence of high technology being used with infant as confirmation that their child was receiving the best possible care, and they watch the monitors as a way of seeking additional reassurances that all was well with their infant irrespective of their understanding of the technology [97].

The language healthcare providers use to communicate with parents about their infant's care and treatment can be impactful. Studies have detailed the effect upon families of un-stated assumptions and values of healthcare providers [98–100]. Fenwick and colleagues [101] explored how NICU nurses behaviour impacted upon parents (mothers). Facilitative nursing behaviours tended to use emotionally and psychologically supportive humanistic language that enabled social connectivity. In contrast, inhibitive nursing behaviours had the opposite effect and tended to use medical-technological words without explanation, which they suggest served to position the nurse as expert and undermine parental status [101].

Timely, emotionally, and psychologically supportive communications are dependably highlighted in the neonatal parenthood literature as important elements for creating positive parental relationships [98, 99, 102–104]. In response, family-integrated models of care (e.g., [105]) universally emphasise partnership working through honest communication and establishing trustful relationships between healthcare providers and parents. However, some researchers have questioned the reciprocity and balance of such relationships as healthcare staff often retain the 'expert role' [96] (Text Box 3.8).

Text Box 3.8 Practice Point: Being Mindful and Sensitive

Nurses and healthcare providers working in NICUs need to be mindful that parents can find the presence of technology both frightening and reassuring.

- They need to factor this apparent contradiction into the words and language they use when communicating with parents, particularly when conveying complex information.
- It is important to appreciate that not all parents will want the same level of detail or technical explanation, though this situation might change over time.

When talking with parents and other family members, try to interpret their verbal and non-verbal communication cues and if in doubt ask them about their expectations and about the level of explanatory detail they want.

3.6   Concluding Remarks

This chapter has highlighted some of the major contributions that health technologies when applied to vascular access have made for improved user and patient safety, the success of vascular access, and improved patient care satisfaction. Health technologies play a vital role in vascular preassessment, aiding vessel selection and optimising procedural and patient outcomes. The application of advanced material and design technology for the manufacturer of vascular access devices has brought about significant patient benefits. Point-of-care ultrasound (POCUS) offers real-time visualisation of the vasculature and catheter during insertion, whilst ECG-guided insertions help identify optimal catheter tip placement. Near-infrared (NIR) holds promise in further refining vascular assessment before insertion. Whilst touch–look–compare (TLC) used in combination with optical sensor technology can provide objective data to support decision-making. However, it is essential that any healthcare provider using any technological aid undergoes a period of education, training, and reorientation to ensure that they are competent and fully conversant with the technology to ensure proper use and avoid compromising patient safety.

Key Points
- Healthcare technology makes fundamental contributions to improved patient safety, better treatments, and health outcomes.
- Select vascular access devices made from materials and designs with proven benefits that best suit the infant's condition, procedural and therapeutic requirements.
- Choose advanced adjunct components and infusion devices for vascular access that match patients' specific needs and promote patient safety.
- Good prospective assessment of blood vessel health, condition. and suitability is essential for preterm and sick infants in NICUs.
- Technologies such as point-of-care ultrasound (POCUS), ECG-guided insertion, near-infrared (NIR) devices, and transillumination can be readily integrated into practice and improve patient safety and procedural success rates.
- Rapid superficial vein assessment (RaSUVA) and touch–look–compare (TLC) are simple and systematic tools to aid in the assessment of vein health and the recognition of complications related to intravenous catheter use.
- Optical sensor-based technologies can aid earlier detection of peripheral vascular access related complications and possibly reduce their severity.
- The presence and use of health technologies affect parents' stress levels and their experiences of NICU care in complex and evolving ways.
- Healthcare professionals need to remain aware of the effects of their words and language when conveying technical information to parents.

Reflective Activity

Read the following case related to a complication arising from vascular access and consider your responses to the reflective questions at the end.

Sade, a premature infant born at 32 weeks gestation is now day 6 and clinically stable. She is tolerating increasing volumes of enteral feeding of maternal expressed breastmilk and has an n-SPC in place in the left hand, providing supplemental intravenous fluids and prescribed intermittent intravenous medications. Emily is a NICU nurse with 2 years of experience and is responsible for assessing the catheter insertion site using the 'touch–look–compare (TLC)' mnemonic to identify any issues with the insertion site. On one inspection, she noted that the site was less soft than before but was reassured that there was no evident swelling and both limbs continued to look similar. Some 40 min later, Emily's attention was drawn by a colleague to a marked swelling around the n-SPC insertion site. A peripheral intravenous infiltration/extravasation (PIVIE) event was confirmed. The infusion was stopped, the n-SPC was removed. Emily was upset about this event as she felt that she had missed the significance of her observations and caused harm to Sade.

Considering the above case, reflect on your answers to the following questions:

1. If you were the colleague, how would you debrief and support Emily?
   (a) Consider that subtle changes may be challenging to detect consistently, especially in preterm infants with delicate veins regardless of experience, the actions taken and their timeliness on discovery, the limitations, and inherent subjectivity of TLC assessments.
2. What could be done to reduce subjectivity and make observations more objective?
   (a) Think about the possible contributions of standardised education and training activities to improve interrater reliability.
3. What else might be done to improve earlier detection of PIVIE events?
   (a) Consider the potential contributions of using continuous real-time sensory-based technologies to monitor the site and their underpinning evidence-base.
   (b) Think about how you could have involved or provided opportunities for Sade's parents to participate in observing for this complication.

References

1. The birth of the web. https://home.web.cern.ch/science/computing/birth-web Accessed 12 August 2024.
2. Bhattacharyya KB. Godfrey Newbold Hounsfield (1919–2004): the man who revolutionized neuroimaging. Ann Indian Acad Neurol. 2016;19(4):448–50. https://doi.org/10.4103/0972-2327.194414.

3. The Nobel Prize in Physiology or Medicine 1979. NobelPrize.org. https://www.nobelprize.org/prizes/medicine/1979/summary/ Accessed 12 August 2024.
4. Rivera AM, Strauss KW, Van Zundert A, Mortier E. The history of peripheral intravenous catheters: how little plastic tubes revolutionized medicine. Acta Anaesth (Belg). 2005;56(3):271–82.
5. Halliday HL. The fascinating story of surfactant. J Peadiatr Child Health. 2017;53(4):327–32. https://doi.org/10.1111/jpc.13500.
6. Halliday HL. History of surfactant from 1980. Biol Neonate. 2005;87(4):317–22. https://doi.org/10.1159/000084879.
7. Curstedt T, Halliday HL, Speer CP. A unique story in neonatal research: the development of a porcine surfactant. Neonatology. 2015;107(4):321–9. https://doi.org/10.1159/000381117.
8. Hugill K. Vascular access in neonatal care settings: selecting the appropriate device. Brit J Nur. 2016;25(3):171–6. https://doi.org/10.12968/bjon.2016.25.3.171.
9. van Rens MFPT, Hugill K, Mahmah MA, Francia ALV, van Loon FHJ. Effect of peripheral intravenous catheter type and material on therapy failure in a neonatal population. J Vasc Access. 2022:11297298221080071. https://doi.org/10.1177/11297298221080071.
10. Pet GC, Eickhoff JC, McNevin KE, Do J, McAdams RM. Risk factors for peripherally inserted central catheter complications in neonates. J Perinatol. 2020;40(4):581–8. https://doi.org/10.1038/s41372-019-0575-7.
11. Karadağ A, Görgülü S. Effect of two different short peripheral catheter materials on phlebitis development. J Intraven Nurs. 2000;23(3):158–66.
12. Biasucci DG, Disma NM, Pittiruti M, editors. Vascular access in neonates and children. Geneva: Springer; 2022.
13. D'Andrea V, Prontera G, Rubortone S, Pittiruti M. Epicutaneo-cava catheters. Chapter 11. In: Biasucci DG, Disma NM, Pittiruti M, editors. Vascular access in neonates and children. Geneva: Springer; 2022. p. 169–88.
14. Tobin CR. The Teflon intravenous catheter: incidence of phlebitis and duration of catheter life in the neonatal patient. J Obstet Gynecol Neonat Nurs. 1988;17(1):35–42. https://doi.org/10.1111/j.1552-6909.1988.tb00412.x.
15. Kuş B, Büyükyılmaz F. Effectiveness of Vialon biomaterial versus Teflon catheters for peripheral intravenous placement: a randomized clinical trial. Jpn J Nurs Sci. 2020;17(3):e12328. https://doi.org/10.1111/jjns.12328.
16. Chhugani M, James MM, Thokchom S. A randomized controlled trial to assess the effectiveness of vialon cannula versus polytetrafluoroethylene (PTFE) cannula in terms of indwelling time and complications in patients requiring peripheral intravenous cannulation. IJSR. 2015;4(12):1075–80. https://www.ijsr.net/search_index_results_paperid.php?id=NOV152135
17. Mathews R, Gavin NC, Marsh N, Marquart-Wilson L, Keogh S. Peripheral intravenous catheter material and design reduce device failure: a systematic review and meta-analysis. Infect Disease Health. 2023;28(4):298–307. https://doi.org/10.1016/j.idh.2023.05.005.
18. ÖzsaraÇ M, Dolek M, Sarsilmaz S, Sever M, Sener S, Kiyan S, et al. The effect of cannula material on the pain of peripheral intravenous cannulation in the emergency department: a prospective randomized controlled study. Tr J Emerg Med. 2012;12(4):151–6. https://doi.org/10.5505/1304.7361.2012.47855.
19. Vercauteren M, Panneel L, Jorens PG, Covaci A, Cleys P, Mulder A, et al. An ex vivo study examining migration of microplastics from an infused neonatal parenteral nutrition circuit. Environ Health Perspect. 2024;132(3):37703. https://doi.org/10.1289/EHP13491.
20. Foster JP, Richards R, Showell MG, Jones LJ. Intravenous in-line filters for preventing morbidity and mortality in neonates. Cochrane Database Syst Rev. 2015;2015(8):CD005248. https://doi.org/10.1002/14651858.CD005248.
21. Van Boxtel T, Pittiruti M, Arkema A, Ball P, Barone G, Bertioglio S, et al. WoCoVA consensus on the clinical use of in-line filtration during intravenous infusions: current evidence and recommendations for future research. J Vasc Access. 2022;23(2):179–91. https://doi.org/10.1177/1129729821989165.

22. Greene ES. Challenges in reducing the risk of infection when accessing vascular catheters. J Hosp Infect. 2021;113:130–44. https://doi.org/10.1016/j.jhin.2021.03.005.
23. Flynn JM, Larsen EN, Keogh S, Ullman AJ, Rickard CM. Methods for microbial needle-less connector decontamination: a systematic review and meta-analysis. Am J Infect Control. 2019;47(8):956–62. https://doi.org/10.1016/j.ajic.2019.01.002.
24. Centers for Disease Control and Prevention (CDC). Guidelines for the prevention of intra-vascular catheter-related infections 2011. http://www.cdc.gov/hicpac/pdf/guidelines/bsi-guidelines-2011.pdf. Accessed 12 August 2024.
25. Nickel B, Gorski L, Kleidon T, Kyes A, DeVries M, Keogh S, et al. Infusion therapy standards of practice. 9th ed. J Inf Nurs. 2024;47(1S):S1–S285. https://doi.org/10.1097/NAN.0000000000000532.
26. ANTT® procedure guidelines. https://www.antt.org/antt-procedure-guidelines.html. Accessed 12 August 2024.
27. Gillis VELM, van Es MJ, Wouters Y, Wanten GJA. Antiseptic barrier caps to prevent central line-associated bloodstream infections: a systematic review and meta-analysis. Am J Inf Control. 2023;51(7):827–35. https://doi.org/10.1016/j.ajic.2022.09.005.
28. Visscher MO, Carr AN, Narendran V. Premature infant skin barrier maturation: status at full-term corrected age. J Perinatol. 2021;41(2):232–9. https://doi.org/10.1038/s41372-020-0704-3. Erratum in: J Perinatol 2021;41(2):360. https://doi.org/10.1038/s41372-020-0713-2
29. Oranges T, Dini V, Romanelli M. Skin physiology of the neonate and infant: clinical implications. Adv Wound Care (New Rochelle). 2015;4(10):587–95. https://doi.org/10.1089/wound.2015.0642.
30. Sauron C, Jouvet P, Pinard G, Goudreault D, Martin B, Rival B, et al. Using isopropyl alcohol impregnated disinfection caps in the neonatal intensive care unit can cause isopropyl alcohol toxicity. Acta Paediatr. 2015;104(11):e489–93. https://doi.org/10.1111/apa.13099.
31. Hjalmarsson LB, Hagberg J, Schollin J, Ohlin A. Leakage of isopropanol from port protectors used in neonatal care-results from an in vitro study. PLoS One. 2020;15(7):e0235593. https://doi.org/10.1371/journal.pone.0235593.
32. Boissière C, Bacle A, Pelletier R, Le Bouedec D, Gicquel T, Lurton Y, Le Daré B. In vitro assessment of isopropanol leakage from antiseptic barrier caps into commonly used needleless connectors. Infect Control Hosp Epidemiol. 2024;45(5):576–82. https://doi.org/10.1017/ice.2023.285.
33. Rutter N. Percutaneous drug absorption in the newborn: hazards and uses. Clin Perinatol. 1987;14(4):911–30.
34. Vivier PM, Lewander WJ, Martin HF, Linakis JG. Isopropyl alcohol intoxication in a neonate through chronic dermal exposure: a complication of a culturally-based umbilical care practice. Pediatr Emerg Care. 1994;10(2):91–3.
35. Hitaka D, Fujiyama S, Nishihama Y, Ishii R, Hoshino Y, Hamada H, et al. Assessment of alcohol exposure from alcohol-based disinfectants among premature infants in neonatal incubators in Japan. JAMA Netw Open. 2023;6(2):e230691. https://doi.org/10.1001/jamanetworkopen.2023.0691.
36. van Rens MFPT, Bayoumi MA, van de Hoogen A, Francia ALV, Cabanillas IJ, van Loon FHJ, et al. The ABBA project (assess better before access): a retrospective, cross-sectional study of neonatal intravascular device outcomes. Front Pediatr. 2022;10.980725. https://doi.org/10.3389/fped.2022.980725.
37. D'Andrea V, Prontera G, Pezza L, Barone G, Vento G, Pittiruti M. Rapid Superficial Vein Assessment (RaSuVA): a pre-procedural systematic evaluation of superficial veins to optimize venous catheterization in neonates. J Vasc Access. 2022;20:11297298221098481. https://doi.org/10.1177/11297298221098481.
38. Harer MW, Chock VY. Renal tissue oxygenation monitoring-an opportunity to improve kidney outcomes in the vulnerable neonatal population. Front Pediatr. 2020;8:241. https://doi.org/10.3389/fped.2020.00241.

39. Hessel TW, Hyttel-Sorensen S, Greisen G. Cerebral oxygenation after birth—a comparison of INVOS(®) and FORE-SIGHT™ near-infrared spectroscopy oximeters. Acta Paediatr. 2014;103(5):488–93. https://doi.org/10.1111/apa.12567.

40. Abd Rahman AB, Juhim F, Chee FP, Bade A, Kadir F. Near infrared illumination optimization for vein detection: hardware and software approaches. App Sci. 2022;12(21):11173. https://doi.org/10.3390/app122111173.

41. Rothbart A, Yu P, Müller-Lobeck L, Spies CD, Wernecke KD, Nachtigall I. Peripheral intravenous cannulation with support of infrared laser vein viewing system in a pre-operation setting in pediatric patients. BMC Res Notes. 2015;8:463. https://doi.org/10.1186/s13104-015-1431-2.

42. Szmuk P, Steiner J, Pop RB, Farrow-Gillespie A, Mascha EJ, Sessler DI. The VeinViewer vascular imaging system worsens first attempt cannulation rate for experienced nurses in infants and children with anticipated difficult intravenous access. Anesth Analg. 2013;116(5):1087–92. https://doi.org/10.1213/ANE.0b013e31828a739e.

43. Phipps K, Modic A, O'Riordan MA, Walsh M. A randomized trial of the VeinViewer versus standard technique for placement of peripherally inserted central catheters (PICCs) in neonates. J Perinatol. 2012;32(7):498–501. https://doi.org/10.1038/jp.2011.129.

44. Ferrario S, Sorrentino G, Cavallaro G, Cortinovis I, Traina S, Muscolo S, et al. Near-infrared system's efficiency for peripheral intravenous cannulation in a level III neonatal intensive care unit: a cross-sectional study. Eur J Pediatr. 2022;181(7):2747–55. https://doi.org/10.1007/s00431-022-04480-1.

45. Hosokawa K, Kato H, Kishi C, Kato Y, Shime N. Transillumination with light-emitting diode facilitates peripheral venous cannulations in infants and small children. Acta Anaesth Scand. 2010;54(8):957–61.

46. Çağlar S, Büyükyılmaz F, Bakoğlu İ, İnal S, Salihoğlu Ö. Efficacy of vein visualization devices for peripheral intravenous catheter placement in preterm infants: a randomized clinical trial. J Perinat Neonat Nurs. 2021;33(1):61–7. https://doi.org/10.1097/JPN.0000000000000385.

47. Singh Y, Tissot C, Fraga MV, Yousef N, Cortes RG, Lopez J, et al. International evidence-based guidelines on Point of Care Ultrasound (POCUS) for critically ill neonates and children issued by the POCUS Working Group of the European Society of Paediatric and Neonatal Intensive Care (ESPNIC). Crit Care. 2020;24(1):65. https://doi.org/10.1186/s13054-020-2787-9.

48. Barone G, Pittiruti M, D'Andrea V. Ultrasound-guided catheter tip location in neonatal central venous access. Focus on well-defined protocols and proper ultrasound training. J Pediatr. 2022;247:181. https://doi.org/10.1016/j.jpeds.2022.05.035.

49. Barone G, D'Andrea V, Vento G, Pittiruti M. A systematic ultrasound evaluation of the diameter of deep veins in the newborn: results and implications for clinical practice. Neonatology. 2019;115(4):335–40. https://doi.org/10.1159/000496848.

50. Spencer TR, Pittiruti M. Rapid Central Vein Assessment (RaCeVA): a systematic, standardized approach for ultrasound assessment before central venous catheterization. J Vasc Access. 2019;20(3):239–49. https://doi.org/10.1177/1129729818804718.

51. Brescia F, Pittiruti M, Ostroff M, Biasucci DG. Rapid Femoral Vein Assessment (RaFeVA): a systematic protocol for ultrasound evaluation of the veisn of the lower limb, so as to optimize the insertion of femorally inserted central catheters. J Vasc Access. 2021;22(6):863–72. https://doi.org/10.1177/1129729820965063.

52. Ostroff M, Moureau N, Pittiruti M. Rapid assessment of vascular exit site and tunneling options (RAVESTO): a new decision tool in the management of the complex vascular access patients. J Vasc Access 2023;24(2):311–317 doi:https://doi.org/10.1177/11297298211034306.

53. Barone G, Pittiruti M, Ancora G, Vento G, Tota F, D'Andrea V. Centrally inserted central catheters in preterm neonates with weight below 1500 g by ultrasound-guided access to the brachio-cephalic vein. J Vasc Access. 2021;22(3):344–52. https://doi.org/10.1177/1129729820940174.

54. Breschan C, Graf G, Arneitz C, Stettner H, Feigl G, Neuwersch S, et al. Feasibility of the ultrasound-guided supraclavicular cannulation of the brachiocephalic vein in very small weight infants: a case series. Pediatr Anesth. 2020;30(8):928–33. https://doi.org/10.1111/pan.13928.

55. Breschan C, Graf G, Arneitz C, Stettner H, Neuwersch S, Stadik C, et al. Retrospective evaluation of 599 brachiocephalic vein cannulations in neonates and preterm infants. Br J Anaesth. 2022;129(5):e138–40. https://doi.org/10.1016/j.bja.2022.08.006.

56. Suell JV, Meshkati M, Juliano C, Groves A. Real-time point-of-care ultrasound-guided correction of PICC line placement by external manipulation of the upper extremity. Arch Dis Child Fetal Neonat Ed. 2020;105(1):F25. https://doi.org/10.1136/archdischild-2019-317610.

57. Brescia F, Pittiruti M, Spencer TR, Dawson RB. The SIP protocol update: eight strategies, incorporating Rapid Peripheral Vein Assessment (RaPeVA), to minimize complications associated with peripherally inserted central catheter insertion. J Vasc Access. 2022; https://doi.org/10.1177/11297298221099838.

58. Barone G, Pittiruti M, Biasucci DG, Elisei D, Lacobone E, La Greca A, et al. Neo-ECHOTIP: a structured protocol for ultrasound-based tip navigation and tip location during placement of central venous access devices in neonates. J Vasc Access. 2021;23(5):679–88. https://doi.org/10.1177/11297298211007703.

59. Spagnuolo F. Global use of ultrasound in newborn vascular access: RA. CE. VA: implantation and management of complications. J Ultrasound. 2023; https://doi.org/10.1007/s40477-023-00813-4.

60. Yang L, Bing X, Song L, Na C, Minghong D, Annuo L. Intracavity electrocardiogram guidance for placement of peripherally inserted central catheters in premature infants. Med (Baltimore). 2019;98(50):e18368. https://doi.org/10.1097/MD.0000000000018368.

61. Capasso A, Mastroianni R, Passariello A, Palma M, Messina F, Ansalone A, et al. The intra-cavitary electrocardiography method for positioning the tip of epicutaneous cava catheter in neonates: pilot study. J Vasc Access. 2018;19(6):542–7. https://doi.org/10.1177/1129729818761292.

62. Ling Q, Chen H, Tang M, Qu Y, Tang B. Accuracy and safety study of intracavity electrocardiographic guidance for peripherally inserted central catheter placement in neonates. J Pernat Neonat Nurs. 2019;331(1):89–95. https://doi.org/10.1097/JPN.0000000000000389.

63. Xiao AQ, Sun J, Zhu LH, Liao ZY, Shen P, Zhao LL, et al. Effectiveness of intracavitary electrocardiogram-guided peripherally inserted central catheter tip placement in premature infants: a multicentre pre-post intervention study. Eur J Pediatr. 2020;179(3):439–46. https://doi.org/10.1007/s00431-019-03524-3.

64. D'Andrea V, Pezza L, Prontera G, Ancora G, Pittiruti M, Vento G, et al. The intracavitary ECG method for tip location of ultrasound-guided centrally inserted central catheter in neonates. J Vasc Access. 2023;24(5):1134–9. https://doi.org/10.1177/11297298211068302.

65. Hugill K. Is there an optimal way of securing peripheral IV catheters in children? Brit J Nurs. 2016;25(19):S20–1. https://doi.org/10.12968/bjon.2016.25.19.S20.

66. Ullman AJ, Cooke ML, Mitchell M, Lin F, New K, Long DA, et al. Dressings and securement devices for central venous catheters (CVC). Cochrane Database Syst Rev. 2015;2015(9):CD010367. https://doi.org/10.1002/14651858.CD010367.

67. Kleidon TM, Ullman AJ, Gibson V, Chaseling B, Schoutrop J, Mihala G, et al. A pilot randomized controlled trial of novel dressing and securement techniques in 101 pediatric patients. J Vasc Interv Radiol. 2017;28(11):1548–56.e1. https://doi.org/10.1016/j.jvir.2017.07.012.

68. Ullman AJ, Kleidon TM, Gibson V, McBride CA, Mihala G, Cooke M, et al. Innovative dressing and securement of tunnelled central venous access devices in pediatrics: a pilot randomized controlled trial. BMC Cancer. 2017;17(1):595. https://doi.org/10.1186/s12885-017-3606-9.

69. Loveday HP, Wilson JA, Pratt RJ, Golsorkhi M, Tinngle A, Bak A, et al. EPIC 3: national evidence-based guidelines for preventing healthcare associated infections in NHS hospitals in England. J Hosp Infect. 2014;86(Suppl 1):S1–70. https://doi.org/10.1016/S0196-6701(13)60012-2.

70. Mason-Wyckoff M, Sharpe EI. Peripherally inserted central catheters: guideline for practice. 3rd ed. Chicago: National Association of Neonatal Nurses; 2015. https://apps.nann.org/store/product-details?productId=23833137. Accessed 12 August 2024

71. D'Andrea V, Barone G, Pezza L, Prontera G, Vento G, Pittiruti M. Securement of central venous catheters by subcutaneously anchored sutureless devices in neonates. J Matern Fetal Neonat Med. 2021;35(25):6747–50. https://doi.org/10.1080/14767058.2021.1922377.

72. National Institute for Health and Care Excellence (NICE). Tegaderm CHG securement dressing for vascular access sites. Medtech innovation briefing (MIB231). 27 October 2020. https://www.nice.org.uk/advice/mib231. Accessed 12 August 2024.

73. Zhang S, Lingle BS, Phelps S. A revolutionary, proven solution to vascular access concerns: a review of the advantageous properties and benefits of catheter securement cyanoacrylate adhesives. J Inf Nurs. 2022;45(3):154–64. https://doi.org/10.1097/NAN.0000000000000467.

74. HB Fuller. SecurePortIV: indication for use (IFU). SPI-IFU01-1903 June 2019. https://adhezion.com/products/secureportiv. Accessed 12 January 2025.

75. Prince D, Kohan K, Solanki Z, Mastej J, Prince D, Varughese R, et al. Immobilization and death of bacteria by Flora seal® microbial sealant. Int J Pharm Sci Invention. 2017;6(6):45–9.

76. D'Andrea V, Pezza L, Barone G, Prontera G, Pittiruti M, Vento G. Use of cyanoacrylate glue for the sutureless securement of epicutaneo-caval catheters in neonates. J Vasc Access. 2022;23(5):801–4. https://doi.org/10.1177/11297298211008103.

77. van Rens MFPT, Nimeri AMA, Spencer TR, Hugill K, Francia ALV, Olukade TO, et al. Cyanoacrylate securement in neonatal PICC use, a 4-year observational study. Adv Neonat Care. 2021;22(3):270–9. https://doi.org/10.1097/ANC.0000000000000963.

78. van Rens MFPT, Spencer TR, Hugill K, Francia AL, van Loon FHJ, Bayoumi MA. Octyl-butyl-cyanoacrylate glue for securement of peripheral intravenous catheters: a retrospective observational study in the neonatal population. J Vasc Access. 2023;16:11297298231154629. https://doi.org/10.1177/11297298231154629.

79. National Institute for Health and Care Excellence (NICE). SecurePort IV tissue adhesive for use with percutaneous catheters. Medtech innovation briefing. London: NICE; 15 March 2023. www.nice.org.uk/guidance/mib288. Accessed 12 August 2024.

80. Zhang S, Price N, Guido A. Addition of cyanoacrylate adhesive improves the strength of catheter securement and integrity of transparent dressing: results from an in vitro test model. J Vasc Access. 2023; https://doi.org/10.1177/11297298231159177.

81. Hugill K, van Rens MFPT, Alderman A, Kaczmarek L, Lund C, Paradis A. Safe and effective removal of cyanoacrylate vascular access catheter securement adhesive in neonates. Front Pediatr. 2023;11(1237648):1–5. https://doi.org/10.3389/fped.2023.1237648.

82. Hirata I, Mazzotta A, Makvandi P, Cesini I, Brioschi C, Ferraris A, et al. Sensing technologies for extravasation detection: a review. ACS Sens. 2023;8(3):1017–32. https://doi.org/10.1021/acssensors.2c02602.

83. ivWatch LLC. ivWatch® breakthrough in IV safety, whitepaper. 2023. ivWatch-Model-400-Whitepaper.pdf. Accessed 12 August 2024.

84. ivWatch LLC. ivWatch® always there, smarttouch, whitepaper: a smarter way to monitor peripheral IV sites. 2023. Whitepaper Smarttouch—ivWatch. Accessed 12 August 2024.

85. Naramore WJ, Brown S, Schears GJ, Cole MA. ivWatch SmartTouch Sensor: the effect of PIV depth and site. 2023.. ivWatch-SmartTouch-Sensor_-The-Effect-of-PIV-Depth-and-Site.pdf. Accessed 12 August 2024.

86. Doellman D, Rineair S. The use of optical detection for continuous monitoring of pediatric IV sites. JAVA. 2019;24(2):44–7. https://doi.org/10.2309/j.java.2019.002.003.

87. McBride CA, Rahiman S, Schlapbach LJ, Schults JA, Kleidon TM, Kennedy M, et al. Comparing ivWatch biosensor to standard care to identify extravasation injuries in the paediatric intensive care: a protocol for a randomised controlled trial. BMJ Open. 2022;12(2):e047765. https://doi.org/10.1136/bmjopen-2020-047765.

88. van Rens MFPT, Hugill K, Francia ALV. A new approach for early recognition of peripheral intravenous (PIV) infiltration: a pilot appraisal of a sensor technology in a neonatal population. Vasc Access. 2019;5(2):38–41. https://doi.org/10.33235/va.5.2.38-41.

89. D'Andrea V, Prontera G, Carlino R, Di Trani H, Carlettini I, Pittiruti M, et al. Optical detection of infiltration during peripheral intravenous infusion in neonates. J Vasc Access. 2023; https://doi.org/10.1177/11297298231177723.
90. van Rens MFPT, Vijlbrief D, Braun S, Hugill K, van Loon FHJ, van de Hoogen A. Peripheral intravenous therapy infiltration/extravasation (PIVIE) risks and the potential for earlier notification of events using a novel sensor technology in a neonatal population. J Vasc Access. 2023; https://doi.org/10.1177/11297298231185536.
91. Cronqvist A, Theorell T, Burns T, Lützén K. Caring about-caring for: moral obligations and work responsibilities in intensive care nursing. Nurs Ethics. 2004;11(1):63–76.
92. Ionio C, Colombo C, Brazzoduro V, Mascheroni E, Confalonieri E, Castoldi F, et al. Mothers and fathers in NICU: the impact of preterm birth on parental distress. Eur J Psychol. 2016;12(4):604–21. https://doi.org/10.5964/ejop.v12i4.1093.
93. Hagen IH, Iversen VC, Svindseth MF. Differences and similarities between mothers and fathers of premature children: a qualitative study of parents' coping experiences in a neonatal intensive care unit. BMC Pediatr. 2016;16:92. https://doi.org/10.1186/s12887-016-0631-9.
94. Al Maghaireh DF, Abdullah KL, Chan CM, Piaw CY, Al Kawafha MM. Systematic review of qualitative studies exploring parental experiences in the neonatal intensive care unit. J Clin Nurs. 2016;25(19–20):2745–56. https://doi.org/10.1111/jocn.13259.
95. Lakshmanan A, Agni M, Lieu T, Fleegler E, Kipke M, Friedlich PS, et al. The impact of preterm birth <37 weeks on parents and families: a cross-sectional study in the 2 years after discharge from the neonatal intensive care unit. Health Qual Life Outcomes. 2017;15:38. https://doi.org/10.1186/s12955-017-0602-3.
96. Pace Parascandalo R, Hugill K. Supporting early parenting following preterm birth. In: Borg-Xuereb R, Jones J, editors. Perspectives in midwifery and parenthood. London: Springer; 2023. p. 83–94.
97. Hugill K, Letherby G, Reid T, Lavender T. Experiences of fathers shortly after the birth of their preterm infants. J Obstet Gynecol Neonat Nurs. 2013;42(6):655–63. https://doi.org/10.1111/1552-6909.12256.
98. Sakonidou S, Kotzamanis S, Tallett A, Poots AJ, Modi N, Bell D, et al. Parents' experiences of communication in neonatal care (PEC): a neonatal survey refined for real-time parent feedback. Arch Dis Child Fetal Neonat Ed. 2023;108(4):F416–20. https://doi.org/10.1136/archdischild-2022-324548.
99. Gallagher K, Shaw C, Aladangady N, Marlow N. Parental experience of interaction with healthcare professionals during their infant's stay in the neonatal intensive care unit. Arch Dis Child Fetal Neonat Ed. 2018;103(4):F343–8. https://doi.org/10.1136/archdischild-2016-312278.
100. Friedman J, Friedman SH, Collin M, Martin RJ. Staff perceptions of challenging parent-staff interactions and beneficial strategies in the neonatal intensive care unit. Acta Paediatr. 2018;107(1):33–9. https://doi.org/10.1111/apa.14025.
101. Fenwick J, Barclay L, Schmied V. Struggling to mother: a consequence of inhibitive nursing interactions in the neonatal nursery. J Perinat Neonat Nurs. 2001;15(2):49–64.
102. Fenwick J, Barclay L, Schmied V. 'Chatting': an important clinical tool in facilitating mothering in neonatal nurseries. J Adv Nurs. 2001;33(5):583–93.
103. Cescutti-Butler L, Galvin K. Parents' perceptions of staff competency in a neonatal intensive care unit. J Clin Nurs. 2003;12(5):752–61.
104. Brett J, Staniszewska S, Newburn M, Jones N, Taylor L. A systematic mapping review of effective interventions for communicating with, supporting and providing information to parents of preterm infants. BMJ Open. 2011;1:e000023. https://doi.org/10.1136/bmjopen-2010-000023.
105. British Association of Perinatal Medicine (BAPM). Family integrated care a framework for practice. London: BAPM; 2021.

Part III

Insertion, Use, and Aftercare of Vascular Access Devices

Peripheral Vascular Access Device Insertion

4

Chapter Learning Objectives

Upon completing this chapter, readers will be able to:

- Relate clinical practice strategies for ensuring safe peripheral vascular access
  - In relation to preparations before insertion, safe insertion, ensuring exit site protection, and device security
- Evaluate the effectiveness of non-pharmacological measures during vascular access to promote infant comfort
- Promote practical opportunities to facilitate greater parental involvement during peripheral vascular access related procedures

4.1 Introduction

Proper peripheral vascular access device (PVAD) insertion, use, and maintenance are crucial components of neonatal care. The significance, in terms of patient experience and well-being of this pervasive experience can be life altering. Preliminary steps in PVAD insertion include consideration of the need for vascular access and that the peripheral route is the most appropriate, knowing that PVAD has short indwell times and high complication rates [1]. Assessment of blood vessels for suitability, selection of the optimum device, and skin preparation are also important prefaces. Determining the best ways to ensure infant comfort and minimise pain experiences are essential skills for nurses. Opportunities to communicate with and involve parents in the procedure should be routinely factored into these preparations [2–6]. Sealing of the catheter exit site, effective device stabilisation, and dressing are readily modifiable practices that can help avoid complications related to device movement and extraluminal infection [7].

© The Author(s), under exclusive license to Springer Nature Switzerland AG 2024
M. R. van Rens, K. Hugill, *Vascular Access in Neonatal Nursing Practice: A Neuroprotective Approach*, https://doi.org/10.1007/978-3-031-81602-4_4

4.2   Selecting the Appropriate Vessel for PVAD Placement

Selecting the appropriate vessel for PVAD placement affects the likelihood of successful insertion and the incidence of complications. Proactive pre-procedural vessel health and suitability assessments can support measures to preserve blood vessels for future needs [1, 8, 9].

4.2.1   Vein Assessment

The rapid superficial vein assessment protocol (RaSuVA) [9] is a simple yet systematic tool that provides a means to quickly assess the location and health of superficial veins [9]. Doing this will help to rationalise the choice of preferred insertion sites and achieve better PVAD insertion success rates. RaSuVA involves visually examining the infants body using eyes alone or with near-infrared (NIR) aids in a systematic way from head-to-toe. Firstly, on the right side of the body and then the left and in the following order: medial malleolus, lateral malleolus, retro-popliteal fossa, back of the hand and wrist, antecubital fossa, anterior scalp surface, and lastly the posterior scalp surface.

In general, evidence indicates that for superficial veins, transillumination devices, NIR vein visualisation devices, and ultrasound can be helpful for identifying veins, venous anatomical relationships, venous valves, and vessel suitability for venipuncture [10, 11]. Findings from these assessments should be documented in the patient's electronic health record and contribute to vascular access management planning (n-VAMP, Chap. 2).

4.2.2   Difficult Intravenous Access (DIVA)

Difficult intravenous access (DIVA) is diversely defined, and attempts have been made to develop predictive tools [12–14]. One example uses a scorecard to predict the likelihood of DIVA [12]. The tool awards 3 points for prematurity and another 3 for been under 1 year old. Additional scores for vein palpability or visibility (2 each) are added together to give a range between 0 and 10. A score of more than or equal to 4 predicts DIVA. Clearly, by using this assessment virtually, all infants in NICUs would be categorised as having DIVA. Such catch-all tools are of limited utility and have yet to be validated amongst exclusively neonatal populations.

Whilst not all neonates would normally be classified as DIVA by skilled device inserters, their unique anatomical and physiological characters can often make vascular access more challenging. Factors such as small fragile veins, limited vein choices, thin skin, and reduced capacity to cooperate can present challenges. Pragmatically, DIVA can be defined as any infant who requires more than three PVADs in any 24-h period [15]. Being described as having DIVA should trigger further consideration of optimal route and device. For instance, in some situations like approaching exhaustion of suitable peripheral veins or clinical instability, it might be that an n-PICC/ECC or a tunnelled CICC/FICC might be more appropriate [16] (Text Box 4.1).

> **Text Box 4.1 Practice Point: The Significance of Selecting an Appropriate Device**
> A well-selected, access route and appropriately sized and located PVAD based on a sound systematic pre-insertion vascular assessment with due consideration of unmodifiable patient factors and potentially modifiable therapy related factors can:
>
> - Improve patient comfort
> - Increase catheter dwell time
> - Eliminate unplanned device removal
> - Reduce the incidence of complications
>   - Phlebitis, peripheral intravenous infiltration/extravasation (PIVIE)

4.3   Ensuring Safe PVAD Insertion

4.3.1   Skin Preparation

Infants in NICUs are uniquely vulnerable to infection risks. Good hand hygiene, such as the World Health Organization endorsed '5-moments of good hand hygiene' campaign [17] is foundational to reducing infective risks associated with skin breaking procedures [18–21]. Neonatal skin, its anatomy, maturing physiology, and absorption characteristics present complex challenges for healthcare providers seeking to balance effective skin antisepsis and prevent iatrogenic harm to fragile skin. Invariably, this involves compromises being made to maintain patient safety whilst simultaneously ensuring adequate skin preparation that minimises infection risk. Consequently, pre-procedural neonatal skin preparation remains a generally controversial and unresolved topic [22–25].

Effective skin cleansing and disinfection involves the application of solutions designed to kill or denature skin flora. Typical solutions containing alcohol, chlorhexidine, or Iodine in combination or alone are widely used in healthcare settings [18–22]. Their use in neonates carries elevated risks for patient harm. For example, through misidentification, systemic absorption causing toxicity, or chemical skin burns [21, 23, 25–30]. Applying skin barrier products at this time might be helpful to provide additional protection from medical adhesive related skin injury (MARSI) or when there is preexisting skin barrier injury or pathology. However, these products should be used with caution as they can have problematic carrier chemicals and are invariably either not licenced for use in neonates or their application is restricted to certain uses. If used, then their application and the rationale for their use should be recorded in the patient's electronic health record.

In NICUs, it is common for skin disinfection regimes to be determined by patient weight and age to reflect the differing risks posed for individual infants by these two factors. The following two unit-based examples from practice illustrate differing approaches. For infants born at less than 27 completed weeks of gestation use aqueous 0.5% chlorhexidine solutions for skin disinfection and then apply chlorhexidine 2% in 70% alcoholic solution for the small area at the insertion site. Ensure to rinse the area with sterile saline after 30 s and remove any excess. For infants born at more than 27 completed weeks of gestation, use chlorhexidine 2% in 70% alcoholic solution. Alternatively, another guideline suggests using 0.5% aqueous chlorhexidine for infants less than 27 weeks gestation or weighing less than 1 kg in the first week of life and afterwards using 0.5% chlorhexidine in 70% isopropyl alcohol. For more mature infants, 2% chlorhexidine in 70% isopropyl alcohol from birth is advocated.

Evidence advises that the method of application is less crucial than the choice of skin antisepsis preparation solution [30]. However, failing to apply skin antisepsis systematically is problematic and can leave untreated areas. Standardising methods to ensure full skin coverage can be helpful in this respect. Simple actions are more likely to be consistently used and can consist of application using back and forth or circular motions within specified application and drying times [18–20, 30]. Measures to reduce the risks of chemical burns such as avoiding overapplication, fluid pooling, and excessive skin contact time can be readily incorporated into NICU protocols. Ideally do not rinse as this can potentially negate the efficacy of skin disinfectants like chlorhexidine gluconate. However, individual infant risk assessments concerning skin integrity, the risk of chemical burns, systemic absorption effects and antimicrobial efficacy need to take a balanced and pragmatic view.

Clearly, the rationales for these different approaches to pre-procedural skin preparation are open to interrogation and require further study before definitive guidance can be issued. In the absence of conclusive guidance, it is advisable for nurses and other healthcare providers to follow local hospital guidelines for the use and application of skin preparation and skin protection products. These guidelines should be based on evidence-based advice, combined with local assessment of infection risk and prevalence, and healthcare provider welfare (Text Box 4.2).

Text Box 4.2 Practice Point: Steps Involved in Preparing the Insertion Site
Hand hygiene
- Adhere to hand hygiene protocols.
  - World Health Organization '5 moments of hand hygiene' can be a useful prompt.
  - Prepare and proactively support parents to be vigilant and challenge healthcare providers compliance to hand hygiene protocols.

Position the infant and provide comfort care interventions with an assistant.
Use Standard-ANTT® technique throughout the procedure (unless contraindicated).
Apply skin preparation at the insertion site safely, preprepared applicators can help avoid overapplying solutions.

- Adhere to local infection control protocols, guidelines, and care bundles.
- Ensure to use locally approved solutions at the correct dilution/concentration in a safe carrier medium.
- Ideally employ a gentle application technique to minimise skin irritation.
- Avoid excessive application and remove residual solution.

4.3.2   Insertion Techniques

The insertion of PVADs requires dexterity and technical skill combined with careful attention to detail. The technique employed for n-SPC insertion generally involves an 'over-the-needle' technique. In contrast, the insertion of an n-LPC can employ other techniques such as the Seldinger and the modified Seldinger techniques. These techniques are described in detail in Chap. 6 which considers neonatal central vascular access devices (CVADs). Regardless of which PVAD (n-SPC or n-LPC) is used, it is imperative for successful and safe insertion that nurses receive targeted education and training and are deemed competent to perform the procedure before attempting either approach (Text Box 4.3).

Text Box 4.3 Practice Points: A PVAD Insertion Bundle
- Review the vascular access management plan (n-VAMP).
  - Avoid previously used veins, damaged skin, veins reserved for central access.
- Provide explanations, guidance, and support for the parents, if present.
- Gather all equipment, ideally using a standardised insertion kit and prepare the environment.
  - Ensure adequate lighting, reduced noise, and foot traffic, for example.
- Position the infant comfortably and administer non-pharmacological comfort measure with an assistant (parent or colleague).
- Perform safe skin cleansing and disinfection.
- Use a Standard-ANTT® or Surgical-ANTT®.
  - Carry out preprocedural risk assessments, including the use of personal protective equipment (PPE).
- Use technological aids (NIR, transillumination, or ultrasound) to visualise the vein and aid insertion.
- Insert the device, confirm vein entry (blood flow at confirmation window), and check patency.
  - See Hints and Tips Text Box 4.4.
- Seal the insertion site with cyanoacrylate tissue adhesive, secure the PVAD likewise, and dress the exit site appropriately.
- Dispose of used clinical supplies and sharps appropriately.
- Document handling and outcomes in the patient's electronic health record.
- Debrief parents or assistants.
- Reflect on your learning in success or failure.

Text Box 4.4 Practice Points: Hints and Tips for Successful First-Attempt Insertion

Use an assistant to hold the infant, or use containment holding. If a parent is present consider using skin-to-skin care.

Stabilise and anchor the vein by gently stretching the skin distal to the insertion site and where you intend to break the skin.

Aim the PVAD at a shallow angle from the horizontal of the skin, often at a slightly rotated angle to vein helps.

– The exact angle for successful first-attempt insertions is highly contextual and requires experience to develop consistency. It will depend on anatomical and device-related considerations. For example, superficial veins and PUR devices often require a lower inclination than deeper veins or PTFE devices, though this is not an exact rule.

As the needle meets the tunica adventitia, a slight change in resistance can be felt; as soon as this tissue layer is penetrated, there is a lowering of resistance as the needle tip enters the blood vessel lumen. In the case of PUR catheters, which are exceptionally sharp, the typical resistance felt during insertion may not be present. These catheters should be inserted at a lower angle right from the start.

Advance the needle and catheter very slowly until you see a backflow of blood into the visualisation chamber. Then, lower the angle if needed and gently advance the needle and catheter further into the vein. Thereafter, advance the catheter whilst simultaneously slowly withdrawing the steel needle from the catheter.

Do not fully withdraw the steel until you have secured the catheter in place.

Do not overapply cyanoacrylate tissue adhesive, only 1–2 drops are required, overapplication will delay curing and create a larger adhesive plaque.

Using remainder glue to add additional securement for the dressing and the edges can prolong its adherence and remove the need for dressing changes.

Avoid using adhesive removers containing harsh chemicals (e.g., alcohol, acetone).

Ensure your familiarity with the design features, weight, and handling characteristics of the PVAD you intend to use.

Know When To Stop.

4.3.3 Preventing Pain and Promoting Comfort during PVAD Insertion

For most parents, parenthood in an NICU is unfamiliar, novel, and unplanned for event in their lives [31]. Parents of infants in NICU, particularly those with preterm born infants seem to have a different experience when compared to those whose infant was healthy and born at term gestation [31]. An extensive body of parenting research and reviews from across the world using different research designs over many years consistently draws attention to the relationship between preterm infant parenthood and high levels of acute and enduring stress. See, for example, [32–50], for an inclusive but incomplete coverage of the available literature.

Evidence (e.g., [31, 34, 37, 38, 43, 49, 50]) and experience concur that emotional and psychological stress in parents can have significant effects on the vascular access process. Increased parental stress levels can influence decision-making, communication with healthcare providers, and their ability to provide emotional support for their infant and each other. Addressing parental stress and providing adequate education and support can contribute to a more positive and collaborative vascular access experience.

Concerns from parents over their infant's vulnerabilities and having feelings of wanting to protect them from pain and harm are ever present. Procedural pain is a common feature of infant experiences in the NICU, some estimates suggest up to 17 times per day [51]. Pain increases heart rate, blood pressure (related to peripheral vasoconstriction), and cortisol levels, impacting cerebral blood flow patterns. Repetitive episodes of exposure to pain and stress experiences in early life affect the developing infant brain and neurodevelopment in numerous profound and not fully understood ways [51–57].

There are few pharmacological measures that are suitable for relieving the acute pain associated with vascular access. In paediatrics, skin numbing sprays and topical analgesia creams based on lidocaine/prilocaine mixes (e.g., eutectic mixture of local anaesthetic—EMLA®) are common. However, concerns about unpredictable skin absorption profiles in preterm and newborn skin largely preclude their use in NICUs.

Kangaroo mother care, (KMC), kangaroo care (KC), and skin-to-skin contact are a group of complementary and overlapping interventions which are variously defined and implemented in practice [58]. Robust evidence supports the view that early and prolonged parent–infant contact through KMC, KC, and skin-to-skin contact has considerable beneficial effects on parents and their infant's well-being [58–61]. These benefits include greater infant physiological stability and improved developmental outcomes, reduced behavioural reactivity to painful procedures, more breastfeeding, more opportunities for parent–infant interaction, and the formation of affectional bonds (attachment and bonding) [59–61]. There is some evidence that some of these beneficial effects are enduring lasting into young adult life [62]. KMC and skin-to-skin contact form one of a range of non-pharmacological interventions aimed at reducing infant pain experience [61–64].

Non-pharmacological interventions focus on creating a soothing, emotionally supportive and more therapeutic environment often using infant behavioural cues to guide practice. Techniques such as administering sucrose solution, breastmilk, or breastfeeding combined with non-nutritive sucking, skin-to-skin contact, and various forms of tactile (positive touch, containment holding, affectional touch), auditory (music, human voice), and olfactory stimuli (mother's expressed breastmilk and body odour) can help alleviate stress and provide comfort. Furthermore, such measures can provide opportunities for promoting parental presence and involvement in care activities like vascular access [65, 66].

Research into the effectiveness of individual and combined non-pharmacological measures has been conducted [e.g., [61, 67–80]. Individual studies show favourable effects on pain scores, infant behaviour, blood oxygenation or other vital sign stability, and chemical measures of stress [e.g., [67, 69, 71–80]. However, most studies and reviews of studies concerning non-pharmacological interventions are affected by methodological weaknesses. The reliability of evidence from these studies is invariably ranked from very low to low, or occasionally moderate quality in hierarchies of evidence-based practice [71]. Consequently, it is invariably difficult to generalise these findings and reliably transfer them to other NICU settings due to definitional and procedural differences.

Research consistently confirms the beneficial effects on lowering pain scores following skin breaking procedures amongst neonates receiving oral 24% sucrose solutions administered directly onto the tongue or buccal surface 2 min before a painful procedure. How sucrose operates its analgesic effect is not known but might be related to metabolic processes involving endogenous endorphins. Sucrose doses can be safely repeated and their effectiveness enhanced by combining with other measures [64, 68, 74, 75, 77, 78, 80]. Though the use of sucrose is often categorised under non-pharmacological measures in some settings it is listed under pharmacological. Healthcare providers should follow local protocols and prescribing formularies in this regard.

Weng et al. [77] carried out a meta-analysis of 35 randomised controlled trials involving a total of 2134 preterm infants. They examined the effect of six non-pharmacological interventions for pain relief on pain scores, oxygen saturation, and heart rate. The interventions included facilitated tucking, olfactory or auditory or tactile stimulation, combined oral sucrose and non-nutritive sucking, or combined groups of intervention. Analysis concluded that facilitated tucking, olfactory or auditory stimulation, and oral sucrose and non-nutritive sucking, or other combinations reduced pain scores. For oxygen saturation, only facilitated tucking and auditory intervention had statistically significant effect; none of the comparisons affected the heart rate in statistically significant effect. The authors [77] report that based on pain score and oxygen saturation measures there were considerable variations in the effectiveness of different individual combined interventions. This makes interpretation of these results and their application into practice difficult.

Effective pain management during PVAD insertion improves the experience for infants, their parents, and healthcare providers and can possibly impact on long-term developmental outcomes. The range of non-pharmacological strategies aimed at reducing infant pain experience is constantly developing. This reflects emerging research evidence and new ideas about what constitutes ethical and compassionate practice [72]. Generally, interventions that promote greater infant self-regulation aim to create a more nurturing environment and provide opportunities for greater parent–infant interaction feature prominently. However, there is considerable definitional heterogeneity and many of these lack standardised protocols. Figure 4.1 summarises many of the current ideas that feature in clinical guidelines for non-pharmacological

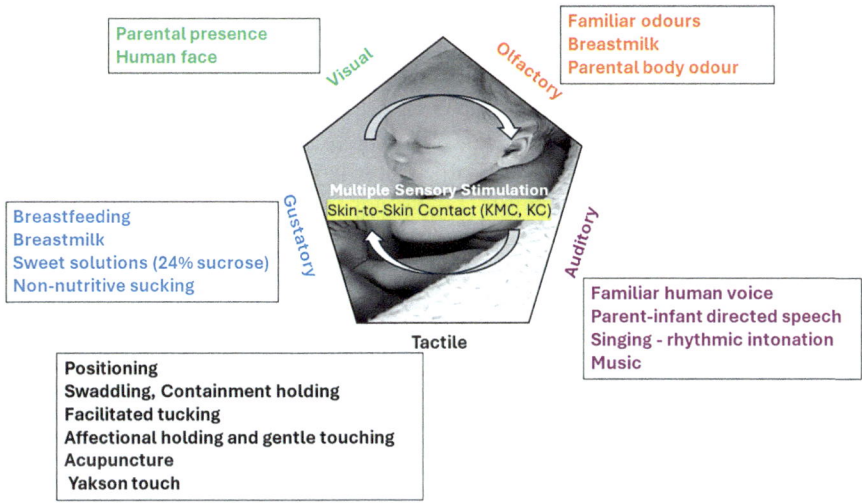

Fig. 4.1 Non-pharmacological interventions that can help categorised by sensory system

management of procedure-related pain. Ideas about the primary sensory focus of these ideas often overlap. In fig. 4.1 the centrality of parent–infant contact is highlighted in recognition of its significance in integrating all the senses.

Proprioception is deeply integrated into the existing framework of multisensory stimulation strategies for neonates. Tactile interventions such as proper positioning, swaddling, containment holding, facilitated tucking, and gentle touch all provide essential proprioceptive feedback, helping to stabilise the neonate's limbs and body. Visual cues like parental presence and the sight of a familiar human face can calm the neonate, reducing involuntary movements influenced by proprioceptive feedback. Auditory stimuli, including familiar human voices, parent–infant directed speech, singing, and music, play a crucial role in soothing the neonate and indirectly supporting proprioceptive stability by lowering stress levels. Olfactory inputs such as familiar odours, breastmilk, and parental body odour also contribute to a calming environment, aiding in better proprioceptive control. Gustatory experiences like breastfeeding, exposure to breastmilk, and sweet solutions provide oral stimulation that soothes and calms the neonate, promoting stillness during procedures.

Central to these interventions is the concept of multiple sensory stimulations. Skin-to-skin contact (KMC, KC) provides comprehensive sensory inputs, directly enhancing proprioceptive development by reducing stress and stabilising movements. Thus, by emphasising how each sensory stimulation method contributes to the neonate's proprioceptive sense, we effectively integrate proprioception into a multisensory framework.

Given the heterogeneity of effect reported by different studies, it is essential to tailor individual or combined non-pharmacological interventions according to individual responsiveness within a bespoke pain-relieving and comfort plan of care. One example from a case study in an NICU in the Netherlands. This article illustrates how with some foreplanning and involvement of all unit stakeholders (nurses, other healthcare providers and parents), a model of parent–infant, skin-to-skin contact during peripheral vascular access insertion was implemented and provides pointers for how this could be done elsewhere [58].

Finally, it might seem obvious and overly simplistic, but the best way to manage pain associated with vascular access procedures is to avoid doing them whenever possible or minimising their number. Taking steps to justify that every painful procedure is essential for patient well-being and that everything has been done to minimise discomfort and pain can positively influence patient and family experience and developmental outcomes.

4.4   Sealing, Securement, Stabilisation, and Exit Site Dressing

PVAD dressing and securement strategies involving tapes, cyanoacrylate tissue adhesives, engineered securement aids, splints, and transparent dressings used alone, in combination, or as integrated systems commonly feature in neonatal PVAD care. Many studies exploring the effectiveness or superiority of different approaches to PVAD securement and dressing are limited to adult or older children study participants. One review of 19 studies (n = 43,683 PVADs) involving patients over 16 years of age tentatively indicated that sutureless securement devices and multi-component approaches might potentially reduce device failure and complications [81]. However, they concluded that much of the evidence in this area of practice is conflicting and uncertain [81]. It seems reasonable to conclude that determining optimal strategies for cost-effective and safe PVAD securement to prevent unplanned device removal or therapy failure requires further development and study.

Specialised securement products, sometimes combined with dressings designed for neonates are available and these can be employed to stabilise the PVAD and keep it place. Examples include the Clik-FIX® (B Braun Medical Inc.), Grip-lok® (Vygon), and 3M™ Tegaderm™ IV advanced catheter securement dressing (Solventum Corp.) ranges. These products often promote that they have a gentle adhesive component. Applied correctly, they can help distribute the forces applied to the catheter, reducing the risk of dislodgment.

Proper dressing of the PVAD exit site is essential for maintaining site integrity, preventing infections, and ensuring patient comfort and safety. Transparent polyurethane (PUR) film dressings with high semi-permeability are commonly used for PIVD exit sites in neonatal patients. These dressings allow for easy visualisation of the insertion site and provide for the exchange of atmospheric gases and moisture vapour, reducing the risk of moisture buildup, which can create an environment conducive to bacterial growth. Generally, PVAD dressings only need replacing if they become loose, dirty, or there is excessive moisture accumulation [20]. If replacement is necessary, follow Standard-ANTT® procedures [21]. Afterwards, document and label the dressing with the date of application. This helps others monitor the dressing's age and previous condition.

4.4.1 Cyanoacrylate Tissue Adhesive

Cyanoacrylate tissue adhesive specially formulated for use in vascular access has become a reliable and commonly used adjunct for securing vascular access devices (see Chap. 3) [20, 82, 83]. The adhesive formulation is widely advocated for securing neonatal CVADs and sealing the catheter exit site [84, 85]. It can also be used to secure PVADs either alone or in conjunction with sutureless securement products [20, 86]. Cyanoacrylate adhesive offers several distinct characteristics that make it an effective choice for securing PVADs in neonatal patients [87].

In the presence of moisture, the chemical quickly undergoes a process of polymerisation forming strong adhesive bonds [83, 87]. Debonding occurs during natural skin exfoliation and renewal processes, but it can be readily removed if required earlier by using a gentle rolling action [88]. Cyanoacrylate adhesive acts as a sealant for the insertion site, this helps to minimise bleeding from the site, and reduce the need for dressing changesdue to moisture build up [83, 87]. Catheter exit site sealing is thought to help prevent extraluminal contamination by immobilising residual skin flora not removed during pre-procedural skin disinfection [83, 87]. This might be the mechanism through which reported reductions in bloodstream infections operate [84–87].

Application is easy, though it is advisable to avoid overapplication which can prolong drying and curing time and reduce flexibility. Cyanoacrylate tissue adhesive can be applied to secure both the catheter to the insertion site and the hub to the skin. This dual securement reduces catheter movement, migration, and dislodgement, ensuring the catheter remains in its intended position (Fig. 4.2). The applied adhesive should be allowed to become dry before applying additional dressings or securing devices. It is possible to add additional drops to the edge of the dressing to increase its adhesion and seal [87]. Current guidelines recommend re-applying an additional 1 or 2 drops of tissue adhesive during dressing changes to

Fig. 4.2 Applying cyanoacrylate tissue adhesive to PVAD catheter insertion site and hub. (Picture courtesy of H.B. Fuller Medical Adhesive Technologies, reproduced with permission)

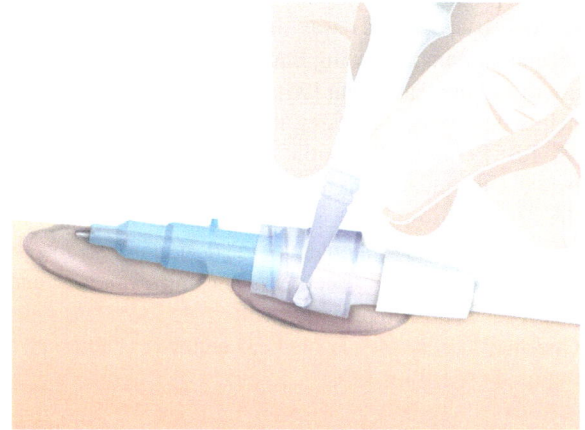

enhance catheter and hub securement, ensuring stability and minimising the risk of dislodgement without causing harm [83].

The first drop(s) seal the insertion site, while the others stabilise and fixate the device.

4.4.2   Splints

Splints or limb boards have long been used in NICUs as part of a strategy to help secure PVADs, immobilise joints, and prevent catheter movement and dislodgement. This practice was argued to reduce the risk of mechanical phlebitis and thereby prolong catheter dwell time [89–91]. Before the advent of commercial designs in the early 1990s, it was common practice to repurpose other medical products such as wooden tongue depressors to make splints on site. These splints were of variable quality, not sterile and were, on at least one occasion associated with infant deaths from highly unusual infections.

Contemporary research data confirming the efficacy of using splinting to immobilise joints or secure PVADs to prolong dwell time compared to not splinting in neonates is not conclusive [90–95]. Most studies report statistically insignificant results in relation to dwell time or the incidence of complications such as mechanical phlebitis, related to catheter movement [90, 91, 94]. Thushara et al. [93] reported that splints improved PVAD dwell time for term infants but reduced it for preterm infants. However, these results were not statistically significant, and the study had several methodological weaknesses [95]. Speculatively, it might be that the perceived benefits of using splints to reduce complications and improve PVAD security might be associated with other unit practices. Differing practices concerning PVAD insertion, securement, dressing, and use likely act as confounding variables masking the effects of splint use in the data.

Singh et al. in a recent review concluded that splinting was not able to demonstrate significant benefits [92]. However, it might be that using splints provides an advantage unrelated to joint and limb immobilisation. The Pepi splint (a flexible silicone based board) was designed in New Zealand to replace existing PVAD securement practice using Elastoplast™ tapes (Beiersdorf AG, Germany) following a serious untoward event [96]. These tapes are known to be highly adherent and can help secure critical devices, though are known to be implicated in serious cases of MARSI [97–99]. The splint was intended to remove the need for direct contact between the tape and skin. Preliminary proof of concept research was supportive of the device's usefulness in preventing MARSI [96]. Further study of the device's effectiveness and refinement of the design is warranted. When combined with newer approaches to PVAD securement using cyanoacrylate tissue adhesive, the splint might prove able to provide an alternate PVAD securement strategy (Text Box 4.5). One that largely avoids medical adhesives, although site dressing would still be required (Text Box 4.6).

Text Box 4.5 Practice Points: Things to Do

Review Requirements

- Ask yourself, is a PVAD a rational choice of intervention for the intended use?
- If not, challenge and seek a rationalised confirmation.
- Engage with parents in decision-making, addressing their concerns and gathering input about their infant's vascular access history, clinical condition, and preferences.

Assess Vein Size, Integrity, and Visibility

- Carefully and systematically (e.g., using RaSuVA) evaluate the size and visibility of the vein, opt for a vein that is accessible, and away from venous valves (use adjunct vein visualisation technologies).
- Ensure the selected vein is free from valves at the tip site or abnormalities like overly convoluted route, thrombosis, or phlebitis.
- Plan to avoid using veins near areas prone to contamination or those that may cause discomfort or excessive movement, such as those near joints.
- Evaluate the condition and integrity of the skin surface surrounding the intended site, avoid areas of preexisting skin lesion.
- Consider the overall health and condition of the infant, noting that some medical factors or fluids might influence the choice of blood vessel.

Prioritise Patient Well-being, Comfort, and Insertion Success

- Be prepared, have everything you will need conveniently to hand.
- Use Standard-ANNT® (rarely are more complex precautions required).
- Implement pain-reliving and comfort measures known to be effective from research evidence or previous infant responsiveness to these measures.

Ensure Sealing of the Insertion site and Effective PVAD Securement and Dressing

- Use 1–2 drops of an approved cyanoacrylate tissue adhesive to seal the insertion site, secure the catheter hub and dressing edges to the skin.
- Use an engineered catheter securement device.
- Use a transparent semipermeable PUR dressing with high transpirability.
- Take measures to prevent MARSI when using medical adhesives.

Ensuring Safe Therapy

- See Chap. 5.

Finally

- Ask parents, what helped to make them feel reassured and involved and what could you do differently next time?
- Ask yourself, am I sufficiently trained, and am I the person most competent to carry out the procedure?
- Ask yourself, do I need assistance? The answer is always yes!

> **Text Box 4.6 Practice Points: Mistakes to Avoid**
>
> **Choosing Inappropriate Veins**
> - Avoid selecting veins that are too small, too deep, or compromised by existing issues. Failing to thoroughly pre-assess can lead to poor vein selection.
> - *Do not* probe or 'dig' for a vein if you miss it or cannot visualise it.
>
> **Having Multiple Attempts**
> - Repeated attempts will cause pain and distress, increase the risk of infection, and damage the vasculature. Minimise the number of insertion attempts by getting it right first time.
> - Underestimating the difficulties of PVAD insertion.
> - Overestimating personal ability and failing to 'step back' and refer to more experienced colleagues.
> - Not intervening (sensitively and considerately) when you see this happening.
>
> **Neglecting Parental Involvement**
> - Failing to involve parents in decision-making and procedural steps can lead to dissatisfaction, misunderstandings, erosion of trust, and complaints.
>
> **Poor Infection Control Measures Compliance**
> - Taking shortcuts over infection prevention and control protocols for expediency.
> - Overly interventionist approach towards unnecessary routine dressing changes.
>
> **Using Larger Veins**
> - Whilst many larger veins could be suitable for PVAD insertion, they are generally not recommended for this purpose in NICU patients being reserved for future n-PICC/ECC insertion.

4.5 Concluding Remarks

This chapter has considered one of the most frequently experienced invasive procedures seen in NICUs, and one that is linked to the highest complication rates. Successful peripheral infusion therapy involves selection of the most appropriate blood vessel and device. Ideas about skin preparation before using Standard-ANTT® led insertion were explored and highlighted unresolved issues. Essentially these issues are encapsulated by a need to balance best infection control measures with the need to prevent iatrogenic harm. PVAD insertion requires skill supported by education, a period of guided practice, and competence acquisition. Vascular access invariably involves some pain. Painful experiences are known to adversely affect infant well-being and development. Considerable effort to reduce pain and promote patent comfort is spent during PVAD insertion. These measures involve a wide range of sensory modifying interventions. Measures that can be readily adapted for parents to deliver and improve their engagement in care. Effective sealing of the insertion site and device securement using cyanoacrylate adhesive can help to reduce the number of complications.

Key Points
- Neonatal peripheral vascular access requires nurses and other healthcare providers to have an advanced knowledge base and demonstrate considerable dexterity and proficiency in practice.
- Rapid superficial vein assessment (RaSUVA) is a simple and systematic tool that can aid in the assessment of vein health and identification of veins suitable for venipuncture.
- Pre-procedural skin disinfection practice requires a balanced approach that considers best evidence-based infection prevention regimes with the need to prevent iatrogenic skin injury.
  - Optimal practice in this area for neonates is unresolved but current ideas support individually tailored approaches using age, gestational age, weight, and skin barrier integrity to guide safe use of chemical disinfectants.
- PVAD insertion is associated with a range of complications that are frequent in occurrence and problematical in terms of infant well-being and outcomes.
  - Nurses need to be proactive in their practices and vigilant in their insertion technique to prevent these complications.
  - Parents who are made aware of what to observe for can better advocate for their infant and add an additional layer of protection.
- PVAD insertion is painful and invariably stressful. Using pain relief and comfort measures is an essential aspect of ethical and compassionate vascular access.
  - Strong research evidence suggests that non-pharmacological measures such as oral sucrose combined with, and without non-nutritive sucking, KMC and skin-to-skin contact are effective at reducing pain reactivity behaviour and stress in infants. Other measures are supported by lower quality evidence but show promise.
  - Parents are well placed to provide stress and pain-reducing interventions, and their involvement can be beneficial for their infant's and their own well-being.
- Cyanoacrylate tissue adhesive is useful for securing PVADs and sealing catheter exit sites, reducing complications associated with catheter movement and extraluminal microorganism ingress into the vasculature.

Reflective Activity

Read the following case related to a complication arising from vascular access and consider your responses to the reflective questions at the end.

Riley, born at 30 weeks gestation is now 4 days old. He was admitted to the neonatal intensive care unit (NICU) due to neonatal respiratory distress syndrome (NRDS). This condition is now resolving, but Riley continues to receive intravenous fluids and medications. During one inspection of the n-SPC insertion site Sarah, the bedside nurse noticed signs of phlebitis. This was thought likely due to mechanical causes due to catheter movement. A decision to remove and replace the n-SPC in a new location was made. After removal, his skin appeared red and had visible epidermal damage that aligned with where securement tapes had been. Riley's parents expressed concern that he might be in pain and that the marks on his skin were due to incorrect removal of the tape securing the n-SPC.

Considering the above case and your reading in this chapter, reflect on your answers to the following questions:

1. How would you answer Riley's parents' concerns?
   (a) Consider the need for honest and open communication and how you might build more trustful relationships.
   (b) Think about the innate risks for vascular access related complications and MARSI that Riley has and what you have done to mitigate their effects—routine observation of the insertion site, prompt actions on discovering problems to limit their severity, measures taken to prevent MARSI, pain relief, and comfort promotion interventions.
2. What could you have done differently to reduce the likelihood of this complication?
   (a) Think about the possible contributions of alternative n-SPC securement strategies such as cyanoacrylate tissue adhesive, and if informing and supporting his parents to contribute to observation and possibly aid earlier detection of the problem might have helped.
3. What additional parent-led non-pharmacological measures might be employed to reduce Riley's pain and promote his comfort?
   (a) Consider the potential contributions of appropriate multisensory stimulation such as KMC, skin-to-skin contact, breastfeeding, parental presence, use of familiar odour, and parental–infant directed speech.

References

1. van Rens MFPT, Bayoumi MA, van de Hoogen A, Francia ALV, Cabanillas IJ, van Loon FHJ, et al. The ABBA project (assess better before access): a retrospective, cross-sectional study of neonatal intravascular device outcomes. Front Pediatr. 2022;10:10.980725. https://doi.org/10.3389/fped.2022.980725.
2. Kelly H. Putting families at the heart of their baby's care. J Neonat Nurs. 2018;24(1):13–6. https://doi.org/10.1016/j.jnn.2017.11.005.
3. Petty J, Jarvis J, Thomas R. Listening to the parent voice to inform person-centred neonatal care. J Neonat Nurs. 2019;25(3):121–6. https://doi.org/10.1016/j.jnn.2019.01.005.
4. British Association of Perinatal Medicine (BAPM). Enhancing shared decision making in neonatal care: a BAPM framework for practice. London: BAPM; 2019.
5. British Association of Perinatal Medicine (BAPM). Family integrated care a framework for practice. London: BAPM; 2021. https://www.bapm.org/resources/ficare-framework-for-practice. Accessed 12 August 2024
6. European Foundation for the Care of Newborn Infants (EFCNI). Infant and family-centered developmental care. European standards of care for newborn health. Munich: EFCNI; 2018. https://newborn-health-standards.org/downloads/. Accessed 12 August 2024
7. van Rens MFPT, Hugill K, Mahmah MA, Bayoumi M, Francia ALV, Garcia KLP, et al. Evaluation of unmodifiable and potentially modifiable factors affecting peripheral intravenous device-related complications in neonates: a retrospective observational study. BMJ Open. 2021;11(9):e047788. https://doi.org/10.1136/bmjopen-2020-047788.
8. Fiorini J, Venturini G, Conti F, Funaro E, Caruso R, Kangasniemi M, et al. Vessel health and preservation: an integrative review. J Clin Nurs. 2019;28(7–8):1039–49. https://doi.org/10.1111/jocn.14707.
9. D'Andrea V, Prontera G, Pezza L, Barone G, Vento G, Pittiruti M. Rapid superficial vein assessment (RaSuVA): a pre-procedural systematic evaluation of superficial veins to optimize venous catheterization in neonates. J Vasc Access. 2022;20:11297298221098481. https://doi.org/10.1177/11297298221098481.
10. Abd Rahman AB, Juhim F, Chee FP, Bade A, Kadir F. Near infrared illumination optimization for vein detection: hardware and software approaches. App Sci. 2022;12(21):11173. https://doi.org/10.3390/app122111173.
11. Curtis S, Craig W, Logue E, Vandermeer B, Hanson A, Klassen TP. Ultrasound or near-infrared vascular imaging to guide peripheral intravenous catheterization in children: a pragmatic randomized controlled trial. Can Med Ass J. 2015;187(8):563–70. https://doi.org/10.1503/cmaj.141012.
12. Petroski A, Frisch A, Joseph N, Carlson JN. Predictors of difficult pediatric intravenous access in a community emergency department. J Vasc Access. 2015;16(6):521–6. https://doi.org/10.5301/jva.5000411.
13. Lee SU, Jung JY, Ham EM, Wang SW, Park JW, Hwang S, et al. Factors associated with difficult intravenous access in the pediatric emergency department. J Vasc Access. 2020;21(2):180–5. https://doi.org/10.1177/1129729819865709.
14. Al-Awaisi H, Al-Harthy S, Jeyaseelan L. Prevalence and factors affecting difficult intravenous access in children in Oman: a cross-sectional study. Oman Med J. 2022;37(4):e397. https://doi.org/10.5001/omj.2022.76.
15. van Rens MFPT, Hugill K, van der Lee R, Francia ALV, van Loon FHJ, Bayoumi MAA. Comparing conventional and modified Seldinger techniques using a -micro-insertion kit for PICC placement in neonates: a retrospective cohort study. Front Pediatr. 2024;12 https://doi.org/10.3389/fped.2024.1395395.
16. Barone G, D'Andrea V, Ancora G, Cresi F, Maggio L, Capasso A, et al. The neonatal DAV-expert algorithm: a GAVeCeLT/GAVePed consensus for the choice of the most appropriate venous access in newborns. Eur J Pediatr. 2023;182(8):3385–95. https://doi.org/10.1007/s00431-023-04984-4.

17. World Health Organization, (WHO). Save lives, clean your hands. A Guide to the implementation of the WHO multimodal hand hygiene improvement strategy. https://iris.who.int/bit-stream/handle/10665/44196/9789241598606_eng.pdf?sequence=1 Accessed 12 August 2024.
18. Centers for Disease Control and Prevention, (CDC). CDC's core infection prevention and control practices for safe healthcare delivery in all settings. (29 November 2022). https://www.cdc.gov/infectioncontrol/guidelines/core-practices/index.html. Accessed 12 August 2024.
19. National Health Service (NHS) England. National infection prevention and control manual for England, V2.4. London: NHS England; 2023.
20. Nickel B, Gorski L, Kleidon T, Kyes A, DeVries M, Keogh S, et al. Infusion therapy standards of practice. 9th ed. J Inf Nurs. 2024;47(1S):S1–285. https://doi.org/10.1097/NAN.0000000000000532.
21. Rowley S, Clare S. Guidance document. Standardizing the critical clinical competency of aseptic, sterile, and clean techniques with a single international standard: aseptic non touch technique (ANTT®). Mount Royal: Association for Vascular Access; 2019. https://cdn.ymaws.com/www.avainfo.org/resource/resmgr/files/position_statements/ANTT.pdf. Accessed 12 August 2024
22. Bagheri I, Fallah B, Dadgari A, Farahani A, Salmani N. A literature review of selection of appropriate antiseptics when inserting intravenous catheters in premature infants: the challenge in neonatal intensive care unit. J Clin Neonat. 2020;9(3):162–7. https://doi.org/10.4103/jcn.JCN_135_19.
23. Ponnusamy V, Venkatesh V, Clarke P. Skin antisepsis in the neonate: what should we use? Curr Opin Infect Dis. 2014;27(3):244–50. https://doi.org/10.1097/QCO.0000000000000064.
24. Muhd Helmi MA, Lai NM, Van Rostenberghe H, Ayub I, Mading E. Antiseptic solutions for skin preparation during central catheter insertion in neonates. Cochrane Database Syst Rev. 2023;5:CD013841. https://doi.org/10.1002/14651858.CD013841.pub2.
25. Sharma A, Kulkarni S, Thukral A, Sankar MJ, Agarwal R, Deorari AK, et al. Aqueous chlorhexidine 1% versus 2% for neonatal skin antisepsis: a randomised non-inferiority trial. Arch Dis Child Fetal Neonat Ed. 2021;106(6):643–8. https://doi.org/10.1136/archdischild-2020-321174.
26. Chapman A, Aucott S, Milstone A. Safety of chlorhexidine gluconate used for skin antisepsis in the preterm infant. J Perinatol. 2012;32(1):4–9. https://doi.org/10.1038/jp.2011.14.
27. Mannan K, Chow P, Lissauer T, Godambe S. Mistaken identity of skin cleansing solution leading to extensive chemical burns in an extremely preterm infant. Acta Paediatr. 2007;96(10):1536–7. https://doi.org/10.1111/j.1651-2227.2007.00376.x.
28. Lashkari HP, Chow P, Godambe S. Aqueous 2% chlorhexidine-induced chemical burns in an extremely premature infant. Arch Dis Child Fetal Neonat Ed. 2012;97(1):F64. https://doi.org/10.1136/adc.2011.215145.
29. Aitken J, Williams FL. A systematic review of thyroid dysfunction in preterm neonates exposed to topical iodine. Arch Dis Child Fetal Neonat Ed. 2014;99(1):F21–8. https://doi.org/10.1136/archdischild-2013-303799.
30. National Institute for Health and Care Excellence, (NICE). Surgical site infections: prevention and treatment. NICE guideline [NG125]. London: NICE; 2019:2020. www.nice.org.uk/guidance/ng125. Accessed 12 August 2024.
31. Hugill K. Father's emotional experiences in a neonatal unit; the effects of familiarity on ethnographic field work. In: Dykes F, Flacking R, editors. Ethnographic research in maternal and child health. London: Routledge; 2016. p. 140–56.
32. Crosse VM. The preterm baby and other babies of low birth weight. 7th ed. Edinburgh: Churchill Livingstone; 1971.
33. Richards MPM. Possible effects of early separation on later development of children: a review. In: Brindlecombe FSW, Richards MPM, Roberton NRC, editors. Separation and special care baby units: clinics in developmental medicine (68). London: Heinemann; 1978. p. 12–32.
34. Moon Y, Koo HY. Parental role stress and perception of the newborn in mothers of preterm babies. J Korean Acad Nurs. 1999;29:174–82. https://doi.org/10.4040/JKAN.1999.29.1.174.

35. Doering LV, Dracup K, Moser D. Comparison of psychosocial adjustment of mothers and fathers of high-risk infants in the neonatal intensive care unit. J Perinatol. 1999;19(2):132–7.

36. Cohen M. Sent before my time: a child psychotherapist's view of life on a neonatal intensive care unit. London: Karnac; 2003.

37. Holditch-Davis D, Bartlett TR, Blickman AL, Miles MS. Posttraumatic stress symptoms in mothers of premature infants. J Obst Gynecol Neonat Nurs. 2003;32(2):161–71. https://doi.org/10.1177/0884217503252035.

38. Franck LS, Cox S, Allen A, Winter I. Measuring neonatal intensive care unit-related stress. J Adv Nurs. 2005;49:608–15. https://doi.org/10.1111/j.1365-2648.2004.03336.x.

39. Orapiriyakul R, Jirapaet V, Rodcumdee B. Struggling to get connected: the process of maternal attachment to the preterm infant in the neonatal intensive care unit. Thai J Nurs Res. 2007;11:251–63.

40. Aagaard H, Hall EO. Mothers' experiences of having a preterm infant in the neonatal care unit: a meta-synthesis. J Pediatr Nurs. 2008;3:e26–36. https://doi.org/10.1016/j.pedn.2007.02.003.

41. Cleveland LM. Parenting in the neonatal intensive care unit. J Obstet Gynecol Neonat Nurs. 2008;37(6):666–91.

42. Obeidat HM, Bond EA, Callister LC. The parental experience of having an infant in the newborn intensive care unit. J Perinat Educ. 2009;18(3):23–9. https://doi.org/10.1624/105812409X461199.

43. Zelkowitz P, Papageorgiou A, Bardin C, Wang T. Persistent maternal anxiety affects the interaction between mothers and their very low birthweight children at 24 months. Early Human Dev. 2009;85(1):51–8.

44. Treyvaud K. Parent and family outcomes following very preterm or very low birth weight birth: a review. Sem Fetal Neonat Med. 2014;19(2):131–5. https://doi.org/10.1016/j.siny.2013.10.008.

45. Magliyah AF, Razzak MI. The parents' perception of nursing support in their neonatal intensive care unit (NICU) experience. Int J Adv Computer Sci Applic. 2015;6(2):153–8. https://doi.org/10.14569/IJACSA.2015.060222.

46. Al Maghaireh DF, Abdullah KL, Chan CM, Piaw CY, Al Kawafha MM. Systematic review of qualitative studies exploring parental experiences in the neonatal intensive care unit. J Clin Nurs. 2016;25(19–20):2745–56. https://doi.org/10.1111/jocn.13259.

47. Provenzi L, Barello S, Fumagalli M, Graffigna G, Sirgiovanni I, Savarese M, et al. A comparison of maternal and paternal experiences of becoming parents of a very preterm infant. J Obstet Gynecol Neonat Nurs. 2016;45(4):528–41. https://doi.org/10.1016/j.jogn.2016.04.004.

48. Pinar A, Erbaba A, Pinar G, Tosun H. Experiences of new mothers with premature babies in neonatal care units: a qualitative study. J Neonat Nurs Prac. 2020;3(1):381 https://doi.org/10.36959/545/381.

49. Bua J, Dalena P, Mariani I, Giradelli M, Ermacora M, Manzon U, et al. Parental stress, depression, anxiety and participation in care in neonatal intensive care unit: a cross-sectional study in Italy comparing mothers versus fathers. BMJ Paediatr Open. 2024;8:e002429. https://doi.org/10.1136/bmjpo-2023-002429.

50. Cruz MD, Fernandes AM, Oliveira CR. Epidemiology of painful procedures performed in neonates: a systematic review of observational studies. Eur J Pain. 2016;20(4):489–98. https://doi.org/10.1002/ejp.757.

51. Zhao T, Griffith T, Zhang Y, Li H, Hussain N, Lester B, et al. Early-life factors associated with neurobehavioral outcomes in preterm infants during NICU hospitalization. Pediatr Res. 2022;92(6):1695–704. https://doi.org/10.1038/s41390-022-02021-y.

52. Malin KJ, Gondwe KW, Fial AV, Moore R, Conley Y, White-Traut R, et al. Scoping review of early toxic stress and epigenetic alterations in the neonatal intensive care unit. Nurs Res. 2023;72(3):218–28. https://doi.org/10.1097/NNR.0000000000000652.

53. van Dokkum NH, de Kroon MLA, Reijneveld SA, Bos AF. Neonatal stress, health, and development in preterms: a systematic review. Pediatr. 2021;148(4):e2021050414. https://doi.org/10.1542/peds.2021-050414.

54. Nist MD, Harrison TM, Steward DK. The biological embedding of neonatal stress exposure: a conceptual model describing the mechanisms of stress-induced neurodevelopmental impairment in preterm infants. Res Nurs Health. 2019;42(1):61–71. https://doi.org/10.1002/nur.21923.

55. Graham YP, Heim C, Goodman SH, Miller AH, Nemeroff CB. The effects of neonatal stress on brain development: implications for psychopathology. Dev Psychopathol. 1999;11(3):545–65. https://doi.org/10.1017/s0954579499002205.

56. Smith GC, Gutovich J, Smyser C, Pineda R, Newnham C, Tjoeng TH, et al. Neonatal intensive care unit stress is associated with brain development in preterm infants. Ann Neurol. 2011;70(4):541–9. https://doi.org/10.1002/ana.22545.

57. Vinall J, Miller SP, Bjornson BH, Fitzpatrick KPV, Poskitt KJ, Brant R, et al. Invasive procedures in preterm children: brain and cognitive development at school age. Pediatr. 2014;133(3):412–21. https://doi.org/10.1542/peds.2013-1863.

58. Sipkema P, Van Rens M, Hugill K. Maintaining parent-infant skin-to-skin contact during peripheral intravenous catheter insertion in a Dutch neonatal unit. J Neonat Nurs. 2024;30(4):393–7. https://doi.org/10.1016/j.jnn.2024.01.004.

59. Bisanalli S, Balachander B, Shashidhar A, Raman V, Josit P, Rao SP. The beneficial effect of early and prolonged kangaroo mother care on long-term neuro-developmental outcomes in low birth neonates—a cohort study. Acta Paediatr. 2023;112:2400. https://doi.org/10.1111/apa.16939.

60. Zengin H, Suzan OK, Hur G, Kolukisa T, Eroglu A, Cinar N. The effects of kangaroo mother care on physiological parameters of premature neonates in neonatal intensive care unit: a systematic review. J Pediatr Nurs. 2023;71:E18–27. https://doi.org/10.1016/j.pedn.2023.04.010.

61. Johnston C, Campbell-Yeo M, Disher T, Benoit B, Fernandes A, Streiner D, et al. Skin-to-skin care for procedural pain in neonates. Cochrane Database Syst Rev. 2017;2(2):CD008435:CD008435. https://doi.org/10.1002/14651858.CD008435.pub3.

62. Charpak N, Tessier R, Ruiz JG, Hernandez JT, Uriza F, Villegas J, et al. Twenty-year follow-up of kangaroo mother care versus traditional care. Pediatr. 2017;139(1):e20162063. https://doi.org/10.1542/peds.2016-2063.

63. Campbell-Yeo M, Eriksson M, Benoit B. Assessment and management of pain in preterm infants: a practice update. Children (Basel). 2022;9(2):244. https://doi.org/10.3390/children9020244.

64. Pillai Riddell RR, Bucsea O, Shiff I, Chow C, Gennis HG, Badovinac S, et al. Non-pharmacological management of infant and young child procedural pain. Cochrane Database Syst Rev. 2023;6:CD006275. https://doi.org/10.1002/14651858.CD006275.pub4.

65. Balice-Bourgois C, Zumstein-Shaha M, Simonetti GD, Newman CJ. Interprofessional collaboration and involvement of parents in the management of painful procedures in newborns. Front Pediatr. 2020;8:394. https://doi.org/10.3389/fped.2020.00394.

66. Ullsten A, Campbell-Yeo M, Eriksson M. Parent-led neonatal pain management-a narrative review and update of research and practices. Front Pain Res (Lausanne). 2024;5:1375868. https://doi.org/10.3389/fpain.2024.1375868.

67. Dezhdar S, Jahanpour F, Firouz Bakht S, Ostovar A. The effects of kangaroo mother care and swaddling on venipuncture pain in premature neonates: a randomized clinical trial. Iran Red Crescent Med J. 2016;18(4):e29649. https://doi.org/10.5812/ircmj.29649.

68. McNair C, Campbell-Yeo M, Johnston C, Taddio A. Nonpharmacologic management of pain during common needle puncture procedures in infants: current research evidence and practical considerations: an update. Clin Perinatol. 2019;46(4):709–30. https://doi.org/10.1016/j.clp.2019.08.006.

69. Nist MD, Robinson A, Harrison TM, Pickler RH. An integrative review of clinician-administered comforting touch interventions and acute stress responses of preterm infants. J Pediatr Nurs. 2022;67:e113–22. https://doi.org/10.1016/j.pedn.2022.08.020.

70. Carozza S, Leong V. The role of affectionate caregiver touch in early neurodevelopment and parent–infant interactional synchrony. Front Neurosci. 2021;14:613378. https://doi.org/10.3389/fnins.2020.613378.

71. De Clifford-Faugere G, Lavallée A, Khadra C, Ballard A, Colson S, Aita M. Systematic review and meta-analysis of olfactive stimulation interventions to manage procedural pain in pre-term and full-term neonates. Int J Nurs Stud. 2020;110:103697. https://doi.org/10.1016/j. ijnurstu.2020.103697.

72. Pineda R, Kellner P, Guth R, Gronemeyer A, Smith J. NICU sensory experiences associated with positive outcomes: an integrative review of evidence from 2015-2020. J Perinatol. 2023;43(7):837–48. https://doi.org/10.1038/s41372-023-01655-y.

73. Shah PS, Torgalkar R, Shah VS. Breastfeeding or breast milk for procedural pain in neonates. Cochrane Database Syst Rev. 2023;8(8):CD004950. https://doi.org/10.1002/14651858. CD004950.pub4.

74. Stevens B, Yamada J, Campbell-Yeo M, Gibbins S, Harrison D, Dionne K, et al. The minimally effective dose of sucrose for procedural pain relief in neonates: a randomized controlled trial. BMC Pediatr. 2018;18(1):85. https://doi.org/10.1186/s12887-018-1026-x.

75. Bueno M, Ballantyne M, Campbell-Yeo M, Estabrooks CA, Gibbins S, Harrison D, et al. The effectiveness of repeated sucrose for procedural pain in neonates in a longitudinal observational study. Front Pain Res (Lausanne). 2023;4:1110502. https://doi.org/10.3389/ fpain.2023.1110502.

76. Sharma N, Samuel AJ. A systematic review of multisensory stimulation on procedural pain among preterm neonates. Pediatr Phys Ther. 2023;35(3):286–91. https://doi.org/10.1097/ PEP.0000000000001012.

77. Weng Y, Zhang J, Chen Z. Effect of non-pharmacological interventions on pain in preterm infants in the neonatal intensive care unit: a network meta-analysis of randomized controlled trials. BMC Pediatr. 2024;24:9. https://doi.org/10.1186/s12887-023-04488-y.

78. Im H, Kim E, Cain KC. Acute effects of Yakson and gentle human touch on the behavioral state of preterm infants. J Child Health Care. 2009;13:212–26. https://doi. org/10.1177/1367493509337441.

79. Kim J. A concept analysis on the use of Yakson in the NICU. J Obstet Gynecol Neonat Nurs. 2016;45:836–41. https://doi.org/10.1016/j.jogn.2016.07.009.

80. Hoarau K, Payet ML, Zamidio L, Bonsante F, Iacobelli S. 'Holding–cuddling' and sucrose for pain relief during venepuncture in newborn infants: a randomized, controlled trial (CÂSA). Front Pediatr. 2021;8:607900. https://doi.org/10.3389/fped.2020.607900.

81. Corley A, Marsh N, Ullman AJ. Peripheral intravenous catheter securement: an integrative review of contemporary literature around medical adhesive tapes and supplementary securement products. J Clin Nurs. 2023;32(9–10):1841–57. https://doi.org/10.1111/jocn.16237.

82. National Institute for health and care excellence, (NICE). SecurePort IV tissue adhesive for use with percutaneous catheters. Medtech innovation briefing. London: NICE; 15 March 2023. www.nice.org.uk/guidance/mib288. Accessed 12 August 2024.

83. Adhezion Biomedical LLC. SecurePortIV: indication for use (IFU). SPI-IFU01-1903. June 2019.. www.SPIVTraining.com. Accessed 12 August 2024.

84. D'Andrea V, Pezza L, Barone G, Prontera G, Pittiruti M, Vento G. Use of cyanoacrylate glue for the sutureless securement of epicutaneo-caval catheters in neonates. J Vasc Access. 2022;23(5):801–4. https://doi.org/10.1177/11297298211008103.

85. van Rens MFPT, Nimeri AMA, Spencer TR, Hugill K, Francia ALV, Olukade TO, et al. Cyanoacrylate securement in neonatal PICC use, a 4-year observational study. Adv Neonat Care. 2021;22(3):270–9. https://doi.org/10.1097/ANC.0000000000000963.

86. van Rens MFPT, Spencer TR, Hugill K, Francia AL, van Loon FHJ, Bayoumi MA. Octyl-butyl-cyanoacrylate glue for securement of peripheral intravenous catheters: a retrospective observational study in the neonatal population. J Vasc Access. 2023;16:11297298231154629. https://doi.org/10.1177/11297298231154629.

87. Zhang S, Lingle BS, Phelps S. A revolutionary, proven solution to vascular access concerns: a review of the advantageous properties and benefits of catheter securement cyanoacrylate adhesives. J Inf Nurs. 2022;45(3):154–64. https://doi.org/10.1097/NAN.0000000000000467.

88. Hugill K, van Rens MFPT, Alderman A, Kaczmarek L, Lund C, Paradis A. Safe and effective removal of cyanoacrylate vascular access catheter securement adhesive in neonates. Front Pediatr. 2023;11:1237648. https://doi.org/10.3389/fped.2023.1237648.
89. Bilal S. Question 1: does use of a splint increase the functional duration of cannulae in neonates? Arch Dis Child. 2014;99(7):694–5. https://doi.org/10.1136/archdischild-2013-305928.
90. Dalal SS, Chawla D, Singh J, Agarwal RK, Deorari AK, Paul VK. Limb splinting for intravenous cannulae in neonates: a randomised controlled trial. Arch Dis Child Fetal Neonat Ed. 2009;94(6):F394–6. https://doi.org/10.1136/adc.2008.147595.
91. Raghavan M, Praveen BK. Effect of joint immobilization on the lifespan of intravenous cannula: a randomised controlled trial. Int J Contemp Pediatr. 2015;2(4):411–4. https://doi.org/10.18203/2349-3291.ijcp20150985.
92. Singh P, Basu S, Upadhyay J, Priyadarshi M, Chaurasia S, Basu S. Effect of splint application on the functional duration of peripheral intravenous cannulation in neonates: a systematic review and meta-analysis. Indian Pediatr. 2024;61(2):158–70.
93. Thushara NL, Singh P, Priyadarshi M, Chaurasia S, Bhat NK, Basu S. Functional duration of peripheral intravenous cannula in neonates with or without splint: a randomized controlled trial. Indian J Pediatr. 2024;91(8):794–800. https://doi.org/10.1007/s12098-023-04756-w.
94. Serane VT, Rajasekaran R, Vijayadevagaran V, Kothendaraman B. Peripheral intravenous cannulae in neonates: to splint or not? J Vasc Access. 2022;23(3):398–402. https://doi.org/10.1177/1129729821996926.
95. Yadav SS, Patel DV, Nimbalkar SM. Functional duration of peripheral intravenous cannula in neonates with or without splint: a randomized controlled trial: correspondence. Indian J Pediatr. 2023;91:13. https://doi.org/10.1007/s12098-023-04880-7.
96. Harris DL, Schlegel M, Markovitz A, Woods L, Miles T. Securing peripheral intravenous catheters in babies without applying adhesive dressings to the skin: a proof-of-concept study. BMC Pediatr. 2022;22:291. https://doi.org/10.1186/s12887-022-03345-8.
97. Lund C. Medical adhesives in the NICU. Newborn Inf Nurs Rev. 2014;14(4):160–5.
98. Fumarola S, Allaway R, Callaghan R, Collier M, Downie F, Geraghty J, et al. Overlooked and underestimated: medical adhesive-related skin injuries. J Wound Care. 2020;29(Suppl 3c):S1–24. https://doi.org/10.12968/jowc.2020.29.sup3c.S1.
99. de Oliveira MJ, Santos AS, Oliveira AJF, Costa ACL, Regne GRS, da Trindade RE, et al. Medical adhesive-related skin injuries in the neonatology department of a teaching hospital. Nurs Crit Care. 2022;27(4):583–8. https://doi.org/10.1111/nicc.12621.

Peripheral Vascular Access Care and Management

5

Chapter Learning Objectives

Upon completing this chapter, readers will be able to:

- Relate clinical practice strategies for ensuring safe peripheral intravenous therapies.
  - In relation to infusion pump use and the monitoring of PVAD insertion sites for complications.
- Discuss the impacts of infusion therapy equipment factors and contextual decisions for ensuring safe infusions.
- Evaluate the utility of preventative strategies intended to reduce the severity of peripheral intravenous infiltration/extravasation (PIVIE).
  - In relation to touch–look–compare (TLC) and optical sensor technology.
- Critically reflect on the management of peripheral vascular device and use related complications.

5.1 Introduction

Peripheral vascular access for infants in neonatal intensive care units (NICUs) is associated with a large burden of complications related to device insertion and their use for intravenous therapies [1–4]. The significance of these complications in terms of patient experience and well-being is often underestimated [5]. In the most severe instances, these complications can have life-altering consequences for infants and their families [1–11]. The previous chapter focused on PVAD insertion and issues around this procedure including the non-pharmacological management of pain and involving parents. These strategies are of direct relevance to the contents of this chapter and should be applied. Invariably vascular access complications are painful for infants and are a source of additional distress for parents. Like all occasions when care outcomes are undesirable, PVAD-related complications can also be a

M. R. van Rens, K. Hugill, *Vascular Access in Neonatal Nursing Practice: A Neuroprotective Approach*, https://doi.org/10.1007/978-3-031-81602-4_5

source of tension, dissatisfaction, complaint and lead to an erosion of trust between parents, nurses, and healthcare providers [12–14].

5.1.1 Overview

Whilst some complications are predictable and unavoidable, others can be prevented. Taking measures to identify aspects of practice that could be adjusted to reduce the incidence of complications could be helpful [8, 9]. One large observational study involving 12,978 infants requiring intravenous therapy identified several unmodifiable and potentially modifiable factors affecting the likelihood of PVAD-related complications [8]. Statistically significant infant characteristics affecting the likelihood of complications requiring unplanned device removal included lower birth weight and the current weight at the time of insertion.

Potentially modifiable factors affecting unscheduled device removal included the type of PVAD (smaller devices, 26 G had fewer complications), insertion site (those in the hand were less likely than those in the ankle or lower leg to have complications), and the given reason for intravenous treatment (fluids of higher osmolarity and non-physiological pH increased complications) [8]. Whilst their might have been some bias in reporting due to the study's methodological limitations, it did include many participants with complete datasets (1% attrition, due to patient transfer or incomplete data) and produced statistically significant results. These findings highlight areas of practice that could be readily incorporated into guidelines to direct practice and reduce instances of unplanned PVAD removal due to complication.

5.2 Supporting Safe Infusion Therapy

Infused fluids can be delivered using several mechanisms. Gravity fed infusion systems, with or without drop counting sensors and elastomeric mechanisms are not widely used in NICU settings as they lack the required precision. In practice when 'flushing' an infusion line or providing 'stat bolus', it is usual to inject the fluid directly from a syringe into the circulation under nurses' hand control. It is good practice to avoid where possible using small volume and bore syringes as these can exert sufficient system pressure to rupture catheters; many advocate using a 10 ml syringe to mitigate these pressure effects. However, there is currently no evidence-based standard guidance and little standardisation of practice. Nurses are advised to exercise caution during 'flushing' or administering 'stat push' medications to avoid infiltration and in the absence of definitive guidance adhere to local guidelines.

In neonates, it is common to use a combination of volumetric and syringe pump infusion devices to support infusion therapy. Despite engineering differences, volumetric and syringe driver pumps share some common design features. Essentially, these are fluid reservoir to contain the infusate, a propulsion mechanism, a microcontroller to regulate fluid flow, often linked to pressure and flow sensors and software feedback loops to enable a degree of automatic self-regulation (Fig. 5.1).

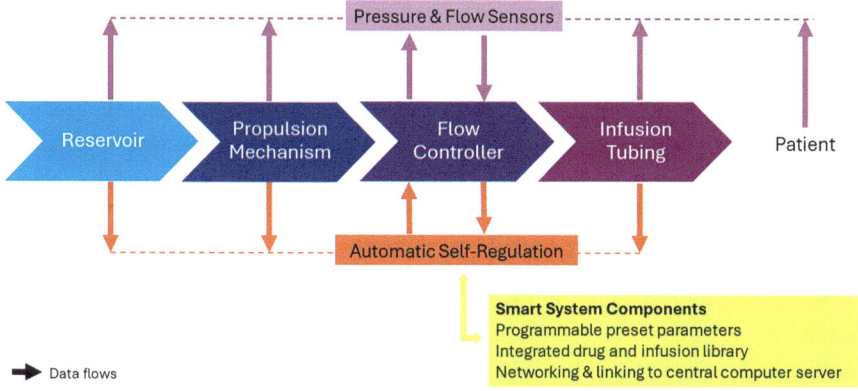

Fig. 5.1 Essential operating principles of infusion pumps

Syringe pumps rely on a piston action using a motor and gearbox to propel a syringe barrel forward and deliver the infused fluid. Volumetric pumps use a peristaltic pumping action acting on a specially designed section of the infusion set to propel fluid towards the patient. These devices are available using rotary and linear peristaltic mechanisms. However, linear mechanisms using a pressure plate and a series of rollers to deliver the pumping mechanism are the most commonly encountered design. Because of the way peristaltic propulsion mechanism generates infusion pressure, these pumps are generally not suitable for blood or other infusions containing biological cells.

All infusion pumps, regardless of their specific design have intrinsic limitations due to engineering constraints and physical science laws concerning fluid dynamics, resistance, and pressure. For example, blood vessel resistance, fluid viscosity, catheter vein size ratio (C:V ratio, see Chap. 4) influence infusion rates and the pressure required to attain them. Infusion pump limitations can lead to clinically important effects and include:

- Fluid/drug delivery delays due to
  - Pump start-up time
  - Pressure displacement in the infusion system—fluid viscosity, dead space in the infusion circuit, in-line filters and one-way valves, syringe barrel and piston recoil, residual infusion line compliance and compressibility
- Inadvertent infusion due to
  - Operator error
  - Bolus administration after releasing an occlusion
  - Effects of pump stacking: height above or below patient level, gravity
  - Flow rate variability: Effects of altitude (atmospheric pressure and gravity) on pump performance, multiple co-infusions into same vascular access device in interlinked pump setups [15–22]

For neonates, the ability of pumps to deliver consistent micro-volume infusions with accuracy is an essential design criterion. The relationship between low infusion rates variations in flow rates is complex [21–24]. Neonates are particularly prone to the untoward effects of start-up delays and flow rate variability affecting the delivery of medications [16]. Flow rate variability can lead to erratic drug dosing and unpredictable total delivered fluid volumes which can have serious consequences [16, 17]. The interrelationship between different infusion components and discontinuous pump flow is further complicated in syringe drivers by the choice of syringe.

Rathore et al. [25] report that differences in barrel and bore size, spring and frictional forces in the barrel, and the varying compliance of different brands of syringe moulding all impact upon performance. At low infusion rates, the effects of these differences become amplified and can significantly affect the time taken to achieve a steady-state infusion rate. One study of seven different syringes operating set to operate at a rate of 1 ml per hour reported that the time to achieve the set rate varied between 89 and 1622 s [26]. In the Schmidt et al. study [27], larger syringes using the same syringe pump tended to take longer to reach target infusion flow rates compared to smaller volume syringes [17]. In practice, attention must be paid to mitigate these effects by careful selection of the type of pump, syringe size, and infusion line priming volume. Generally, the best results, in terms of infusion stability are got from using matched syringes and infusion sets calibrated for use with the infusion pump [25, 27]. However, this might create a need to negotiate a 'tie-in' purchasing relationship with equipment providers.

In an era of economic difficulties and uncertain supply line continuity, some hospitals might be tempted to diversify their consumable medical supply sources. However, such purchasing decisions carry risk. Took and Howell's [28] study implies a degree of caution is warranted. Testing of different commercially available syringes for their performance characteristics under a range of conditions typical of clinical conditions revealed wide and unpredictable variations of different syringe materials and performance. In the worst performing test systems, there was a risk of fluid under infusion of up to 10% and of over infusion up to 24% above intended volumes [28].

5.2.1 Smart Infusion Systems

Medical engineering has over the years sought to improve upon the limitations of existing infusion pumps by developing more sophisticated pumps with higher quality tolerances. Modern syringe driver and volumetric pumps come equipped with a wide range of additional features to help better regulate infusion accuracy and safety. These design features can include air-in-line detection, infusion pressure monitoring, occlusion alarms, user set infusion pressure limits, 'back off' (to prevent inadvertent bolus upon restarting after suspected occlusion), anti-tampering controls, and soft and hard alarm statuses. The current pinnacle of design for neonatal infusion pumps is the so-called smart systems which incorporate arrangements for drug error prevention.

These systems integrate with one another at varying operational levels, have embedded bespoke (to reflect local prescribing practices) drug/infusion library, and can be configured to use locally installed operating parameters. Cross checking against the library can help to prevent infusion and drug prescribing, dispensing or administration errors. However, they are fallible [29] and NICUs should have in place a system of audit and clinical risk management to prevent and act on reports of errors or near-miss medication errors [29]. Smart infusion systems are complex, and staff should not use them until they have been trained and deemed competent to do so.

Root cause analysis assigns medication errors to several fundamental causes. These causes can be broadly grouped into three: (1) lack of knowledge, (2) failure to follow established guidelines and rules, and (3) poor healthcare provider performance. Poor performance is the largest group and is attributed to human factors, including fatigue, distraction, interruption, and workload. Smart pumps increase medication safety, but only when they are used correctly and there are high levels of user compliance with operating software [30].

Schnock and colleagues [31] examining smart pump use in 441 infants ($n = 905$ intravenous medications administrations) reported a lack of compliance in following drug library guidance and correct use of the pumps. Of the 130 errors they observed (rate 14.4 per 100 medications), most were attributable to input errors (5.3/100). The remainder were due to unauthorised entries (i.e., administration not accompanied by order/prescription) or errors on dose entry (06/100). On investigation, 68 errors were deemed not to have caused patient harm and the remainder did not reach the patient.

It is reassuring that the errors were relatively minor in nature, and most were prevented by later stages in the checking procedures. It is unclear from the article if the 'unauthorised entries' are related to poor prescribing practices, limitations of smart pump operating protocols, a delay on the system registering the order/prescription, or some urgency in the clinical situations requiring prompt action on verbal instruction. However, the considerable number of input and dose entry errors clearly raises issues around the effectiveness of staff training and the possible effects of fatigue on staff performance.

Waterson and Bedner [32] conducted an extensive analysis of event logs from 1183 infusion pumps over nearly 7 years (6482 days, Jan 2000–Sept. 2017) concerning four critical medications (dopamine, dobutamine, adrenaline, and noradrenaline). Across the whole hospital site, there were 1.39 alarms per infusion. However, analysis by department revealed considerable variation. Unsurprisingly, given the medications examined, critical areas had the highest incidence of alarms for these four medications. The highest alarm rate was reported from paediatric intensive care (8.61 alarms per infusion). In contrast, the NICU (3.71 alarms per infusion) was the lowest of all critical care areas. Many of the NICU alarms were related to downstream occlusion and this could have clinically significant effects. For neonates, repeated interruptions to the delivery of these medications due to occlusion alarms and delays on restart could contribute to inadvertent over or under infusion and suboptimal therapeutic effect. Reasons for the differences between departments were not clear but could relate to differences in protocols, patient contextual factors, or an inability to set dynamic alarm parameters. Nevertheless, the authors conclude that quantitatively tracking the number, cause of infusion pump alarms, and nursing staff responsiveness could establish a benchmark to inform strategies to reduce alarm fatigue.

5.2.2   Alarm Fatigue

Melton et al. [30] observed that prolonged clusters of audible 'soft alerts' (non-actionable alarms) tended to desensitise nurses to high priority alerts leading to delays in response. This phenomenon often labelled 'alarm fatigue' is recognised as a potential patient safety issue internationally [30, 33–36]. The phenomenon is particularly evident in critical care areas that use a high number of physiological monitoring and therapy delivery devices [30, 32–35]. Excessive noise from medical device alarms contributes to sensory overload and can be directly related to nurse's characterisation of their work environment as stressful [37].

To resolve this situation, many healthcare organisations have focused on delivering targeted staff training to enable staff to better understand the equipment they are using and implementing standardised practices around setting alarm parameters. Medical device design has incorporated features, such as customisable safety limits, multimodal alarms which seek to differentiate visual and auditory signalling for high or low priority alarms, and more recently testing of machine learning algorithms to filter out nuisance alarms. Despite these improvements, alarm fatigue remains an unresolved patient safety issue [38, 39] and nurses need to remain vigilant to differentiate critical alerts from the background. Ensuring that individual team members are supported, not overburdened, and sufficiently rested to be able to focus on their work can reduce fatigue and error. Furthermore, been trained in the use of equipment, having processes in place to set alarms parameters appropriate to the individual patient, and having protocols to manage common situations (e.g., occlusion alarms) can also contribute to fewer patient safety events.

5.2.3   In-Line Pressure Monitoring

Increasingly infusion pumps have incorporated into their body or as a peripheral attachment in-line sensing technologies to measure flow and pressure dynamics. Some infusion pumps offer the option to set occlusion alarms dynamically based on feedback from the infusion circuit. This technology when used to its best can ensure that infants are exposed to lower overall infusion line pressures and has the potential for earlier notification of changes in infusion line pressures. Theoretically mapping pressure and fluid flow can help to detect occlusions and infiltration events [40]. However, the reality in practice is not that simple and relying on in-line pressure monitoring to detect infiltration is imprecise and unreliable.

Infusion line additions such as one-way valves and in-line filters require increased infusion pressure to overcome flow resistance, and this might mask the more subtle pressure and flow changes due to PIVIE seen in infants. Typically, as an infusion pump encounters resistance in the fluid line, it will increase the infusion pressure (within its set limits) to overcome this resistance. If the pressure exceeds to maximum set for a specific amount of time, the pump will then signal an alert. However, in neonates with venous pressure of less than 10 mmHg, what can happen is that pressure will increase but then the vein will rupture, and the infusion line pressure will diminish. Later when the pressure from infiltrated fluid in the surrounding tissue is high enough to cause back pressure though the infusion line, pressure will again increase towards alarm levels. The result is a potentially large volume of infiltrated fluid and no occlusion alarm until the last moment. Large volume infiltration (PIVIE events) or having an extended time before their identification will lead to more severe complications, longer healing time, more pain experience, and might affect staff–parent trust [13, 14, 41, 42]. This is clearly undesirable, and healthcare providers have put in place several strategies to prevent and detect these adverse events earlier, e.g., intermittent 'touch–look–compare' assessments and continuous site monitoring using optical sensor technology.

5.2.4 Managing Occlusion Pump Alarms

Blockages preventing the flow of infused fluids are collectively referred to as occlusions. Signs include resistance to infusion and infusion pump occlusion alarms, which might be an early sign of a more worrying developing complication. The causes can be external such as incorrect infusion pump alarm settings, infusion line trapping, twisting, or kinking and readily rectified or prevented. Internal occlusions refer to when the blockage is catheter related. The cause of these occlusions can be difficult to ascertain. They can include precipitation due to medication incompatibility, improper flushing technique, external pressure acting on the catheter due to limb movement/position or joint flexion, inflammation, thrombus formation, or vascular spasm.

To manage catheter-related occlusion, healthcare providers might reposition limbs and joints, provide gentle tactile stroking of the affected limb, or use a saline flush. If planning to use a flush, it is important to rule out peripheral intravenous infiltration extravasation (PIVIE) as the cause beforehand and secondly take care to avoid inadvertently administering a bolus of medication or a vasoactive/vesicant solution. It is essential to avoid being overly confident about the ease of flushing or blood flowing into the catheter on aspiration as evidence of no infiltration. In cases of severe or persistent occlusion, the PVAD may need to be replaced. Ensuring that pump pressure alarms are appropriate is important to avoid inadvertent and repetitive alarms which can contribute to increased handling, interrupted rest for infants, and alarm fatigue, resulting in reduced responsiveness [30, 33, 38]. Strategies for alarm management are required to reduce the consequences of alarm fatigue and ensure prompt responses by nurses [34]. Figure 5.2 summaries one approach for systematically investigating and resolving pump occlusion alarms (Text Box 5.1).

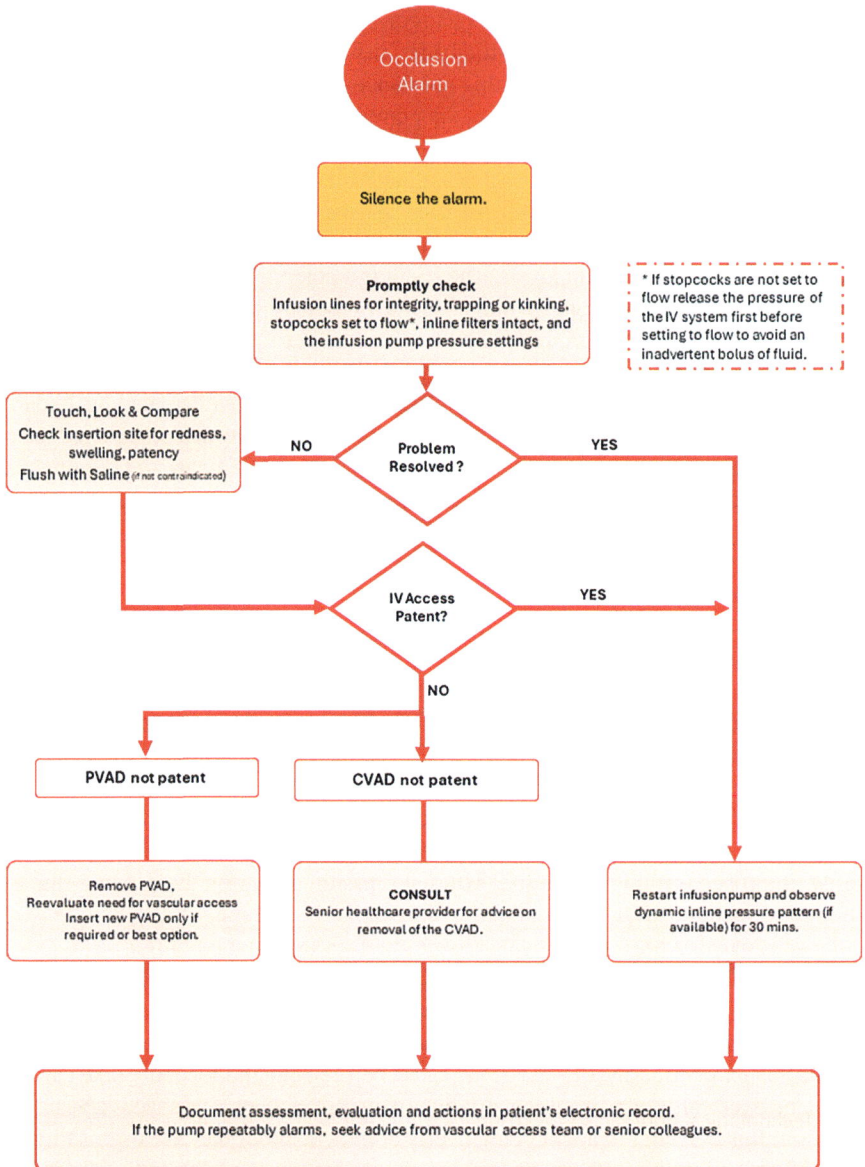

Fig. 5.2 Managing occlusion pump alarms

Text Box 5.1 Practice Point: Safe Use of Neonatal Smart Pump Technologies
- Only use pumps that are configured for neonatal use
  - Do not loan pumps from other departments before having them reset by biomedical engineers
- Select syringe driver and volumetric pump combinations based on appraisal of fluid type, reservoir volume, and infusion rates
- Use standard operating protocols for the different drugs, dilutions, and infusion combinations in use in your NICU, including typical infusion line setups
- Choose syringes with the lowest possible volume suitable for the required infusion volume and dilution
- Select infusion lines with low priming volumes and low flow resistance
- Use the minimal occlusion pressure and time to alarm delay settings that are clinically informative but not so overly sensitive as to generate excessive false alarms
  - Time to alarm alert can vary depending upon programmed alarm threshold pressure
- Avoid vertical displacement of infusion pumps, particularly syringe drivers
  - Take care over effects of pump stacking and siphonage
  - Take care over effects of raising and lowering incubator height to accommodate variations in nurse or parent height during procedures or during facilitation of parent–infant skin-to-skin contact
- Ensure you have undergone a period of familiarisation and training in the use of the smart pump systems and have been assessed as competent to use them
  - If you haven't been trained in use, *do not use.*

5.3   PVAD Complications

International research reports conducted over recent decades consistently highlight that neonatal peripheral infusion therapy continues to be associated with a distressing burden of complications [1–7, 9, 43–49]. These complications directly affect patient well-being and development and are a source of concern for parents and healthcare providers alike [50–52]. Current estimates submit complication rates involving peripheral catheters of around 55%, with some reports indicating much higher incidences of up to 78% [45]. Across all studies, the most common category recorded is infiltration/extravasation representing about half of all cases, followed by phlebitis, occlusion, and catheter dislodgment [1, 9, 43, 44, 46–49]. However, these figures are probably an underestimate as most reports fail to capture other categories of harm such as medical adhesive related skin injury (MARSI) [5, 6, 11, 53].

The categorisation of complications is subject to differing definitions, diagnosis, surveillance, and documentation practices. This situation might explain some of the variability in complication incidence reporting. For example, practice observations indicate that leaks and accidental catheter removals, despite them adding to infant discomfort and stress from handling are rarely documented unless they foreshadow other complications such as phlebitis infiltration or reportable untoward events.

5.3.1 Leaks and Accidental Removals

Accidental removal or dislodgment of the PVAD can occur due to infant movement or through inappropriate handling by others. It is also more likely to occur when infants are unsettled. Effective securement after insertion, ensuring optimal infant comfort, and including information about how best to handle the PVAD and infusion lines into routine parent education can help to limit this complication. Leakage occurs when there is a breach in the infusion system, which may result from infusion line connections, accidental catheter dislodgment, or from around the insertion site. Additionally, if the pressure inside the vein exceeds the pressure generated by the infusion pump, backflow of infusion fluids will occur, leading to leakage. This situation obviously leads to the escape of fluid or medication away from its intended target (the patient's vasculature), resulting in inadequate therapy and fluid and medication infusion error, increased infection risk, unplanned PVAD replacement, or dressing change.

Often the cause of leakage is user error, patient movement, or the wrong choice of device. Clinical observation suggests that it is largely managed at the cot side, unreported as a complication, nor documented in patient medical records by nurses. Regardless, it is essential to identify the likely cause by inspecting all components of the infusion system before replacing any damaged or compromised parts aseptically. Pre-emptive use of cyanoacrylate tissue adhesive to seal the exit site and secure the PVAD can mitigate the risk of leakage associated with catheter movement [54].

Efforts to reduce the incidence and severity of PVAD use and infusion related complications using novel clinical approaches or technological advances often feature in the literature. Interventions often focus on prevention, earlier detection, more informed evidence-based treatments, or a combination of these. An example of two key technological innovations targeted at preventing complications associated with peripheral infusion therapy. Firstly, the widely disseminated low-tech touch–look–compare approach often abbreviated as the mnemonic 'TLC' and secondly continuous monitoring of catheter insertion site using sensor devices.

5.4 Infusion Site Monitoring for the Early Detection of Complications

5.4.1 Touch–Look–Compare (TLC)

The touch–look–and compare (TLC) mnemonic is a structured (Fig. 5.3) though subjective tool for infusion site monitoring conducted at least hourly. If used routinely, it can help to warn nurses about emerging potential complications related to intravenous therapy [7]. This method involves assessing and comparing the

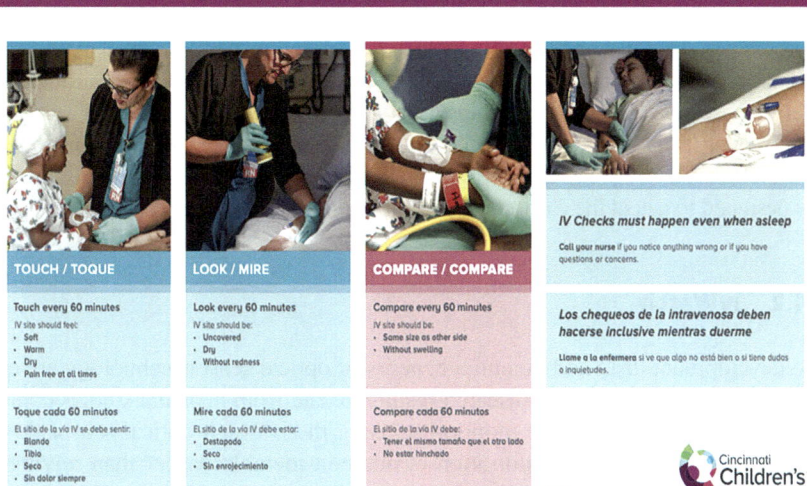

Fig. 5.3 Touch–look–compare. (Image source: Cincinnati Children's Hospital Medical Center, reproduced with permission)

characteristics of the PVAD (n-SPC or n-LPC) site through palpation, visual inspection, and comparison at least every hour [55] (Text Box 5.2).

Text Box 5.2 Practice Point: Using TLC

Touch

- Gently palpate the PVAD site to assess its condition. The site should feel soft, warm (indicating proper blood flow), dry (without signs of leakage), and be pain-free.

Look

- Visually examine the PVAD site for any abnormalities. The site should be dry (without any moisture or exudate) and free of redness or signs of inflammation.

Compare

- Contrast the size of the PVAD site and limb with the equivalent areas on the other side of the body, they should match. There should be no noticeable swelling, colour changes, or oedema.

Document your findings and actions in the patient's electronic health record.
   Act on your findings.

To ensure the validity of the TLC tool and reduce the inherent subjectivity of human-led assessment, particularly in those fatigued, it is essential that a standardised approach is used across a whole NICU. Comprehensive initial and ongoing targeted education, training and competence sign off using simulation, and case scenarios based on real events can help to improve interrater reliability, performance, and consistency of use and interpretation. Parents can be readily included in education to enable them to undertake the looking and comparing components of the tool. Doing this will provide an additional level of observation over the 59 min in between documented observation and could enable better integration of parents into care and shared decision-making. This tool can be complemented by continuous insertion site monitoring using optical sensor technology designed to detect the early signs of infiltration using objective criteria [9].

5.4.2 ivWatch

The development, use, and potential benefits of optical sensor technology are considered in detail in Chap. 3. Research results to date from neonatal studies confirm that continuous insertion site monitoring using the ivWatch optical sensor device can lead to notification of infiltration events considerably earlier than relying on observation methods alone [9, 47, 48, 56], sometimes up to 6 h earlier [56].

Data to hand suggests that when this technology is used to routinely monitor PVAD insertion sites, earlier notification leads to less severe categories of PIVIE. If further data and analysis confirms this, then combining nurse-led TLC and parent observation with this technology might become the new standard for PIVIE detection and prevention of its most serious form.

5.5 Phlebitis

Phlebitis, inflammation of the vein is numerically the most common complication associated with PVAD insertion and use [2, 3, 7]. There are several types of phlebitis, categorised by their causation or trigger (Table 5.1). These categorisations provide insight into the various causes and triggers of phlebitis. Proper identification of the type of phlebitis is essential for appropriate treatment, surveillance, and prevention. Management often involves the removal and treatment of the primary cause, as well as measures to provide pain relief and comfort.

5.6 Medical Adhesive Related Skin Injury (MARSI)

Medical adhesives perform essential functions and solve several problems associated with securing dressings and medical devices for the delivery of patient care. However, when used inappropriately or inadvisably, medical adhesives can create new problems [53]. Medical adhesive related skin injury (MARSI) is a common and largely underreported phenomenon [6]. In neonates, particularly those born preterm with underdeveloped skin barrier functionality, adhesives used in dressings and

Table 5.1 A typology of phlebitis

Infectious phlebitis	Occurs when an infection enters the bloodstream and causes localised inflammation of the vein Treatment typically involves removal and antibiotics to address the underlying infection
Chemical phlebitis	Results from the irritation of the vein wall due to exposure to substances administered through the PVAD Irritating substances can include medications that are too concentrated or too acidic Management may involve changing the medication or diluting it before administration
Mechanical phlebitis	Occurs when the vein is irritated or damaged mechanically. This can happen due to patient movement, PVAD movement due to inadequate securement, insertion of an overlarge PVAD for the vessel size, and PVAD material properties Preventive measures such as ensuring patient rest and comfort, careful section of PVAD device material and size, avoiding insertion in areas of flexion, and effective securement using cyanoacrylate tissue adhesive are helpful
Post-removal phlebitis	Refers to inflammation occurring after PVAD removal It can result from residual irritation caused by the PVAD, infused fluids, or infection Management often involves pain relief and local care to reduce inflammation

tapes have been linked to tissue injury. This includes epidermal stripping, skin tears, blistering or maceration, and contact dermatitis [5, 6, 53, 54].

Treatment is largely confined to measures to ensure pain relief, prevent opportunistic infection, promote skin healing, and reduce scarring. Prevention rests on avoiding overuse and overapplication of chemically harsh or over strong medical adhesives. Ensuring selective use of less harmful adhesives with lower adhesion, avoiding overtightening fixation devices leading to pressure related injury, reducing dressing change frequency to a minimum for patient comfort and safety can also be supportive strategies. Gentle removal of adhesives, only if clinically indicated, and otherwise relying on natural cycles of skin exfoliation to loosen adhesion over time are also helpful. Some practice commentators suggest that the application of protective skin barrier products before applying medical adhesives to the skin might be a useful adjunct intervention. However, their use should be carefully considered beforehand to avoid additional risks from their use.

5.7 Peripheral Intravenous Infiltration Extravasation (PIVIE)

Infiltration occurs when a non-vesicant fluid leaks into the surrounding tissue instead of entering the vein. Extravasation involves the leakage of vesicant solutions. However, both instances can lead to serious tissue damage. Complications associated with infiltration and extravasation are commonly combined using the acronym PIVIE regardless of the nature of the fluid. Van Rens et al. [8] evaluated the impact of unmodifiable and potentially modifiable factors on complication rates in neonates. Of the 12,978 neonates requiring a PVAD in their study, 59% had unplanned removal due to complications. The most common cause of PVAD failure, affecting 40% of all occurrences was PIVIE. This result confirms those found in other studies and in other patient groups (e.g., [2, 9, 43, 48]).

5.7.1 Signs of PIVIE

Signs of PIVIE include localised swelling (sometimes extensive) and coolness to the touch (reflecting the temperature of the leaked fluid rather than infant skin temperature). Redness or pallor around the insertion site, skin blistering or ulceration, hypoperfusion and ischaemia, and tissue necrosis can all feature depending on the chemical nature of the leaked fluid [49, 57]. Prompt action in managing PIVIE to prevent further tissue damage is essential, particularly if the infiltration is extensive or the infused fluid is vesicant or vasoactive. In effect delays in recognition and treatment, 'lost time' leads to potentially greater tissue loss and patient harm [58].

5.7.2 Determining the Severity of PIVIE

Forecasting functional loss or lasting cosmetic damage after a PIVIE event is unpredictable. Although the more severe the PIVIE and the more harmful the leaked fluids are, there is increased likelihood of lasting harm. There are several approaches towards staging the severity grading of PIVIE. Simple staging rules such as ranking the injury between 0 (least harmful) to 4 (severe harm) were originally constructed based on adult data and the assumption that the highest grade is equivalent to the greatest harm. Such grading systems are generally not endorsed for determining individual patient need [7] but can be used for surveillance audits. More detailed assessments tools can help to specify the nature, extent, and severity of injury and guide treatment decisions.

The Cincinnati Children's Hospital approach can be used to measure the extent and volume of the infiltration and assess the risk of potential harm from the infiltrated fluid (Fig. 5.4) [55, 59]. This tool requires nurses to first define the edges of the infiltration and measure the longest dimensions (X). Secondly, measure the distance from the axilla to the tip of the longest finger (Y), a proxy measure of infant size. Using the formula, $(X/Y)*100$ will give a percentage score. This score, used alongside a predetermined colour coded (green, amber, or red) infusion fluid/drug risk categorisation can be used to guide management decisions such as whether to use hyaluronidase or administer phentolamine, for example.

Using POCUS to characterise the nature and extent of PIVIEs has been proposed [60]. Boyar et al. reported on ten infants with severe PIVIE and described a method for using ultrasound to measure the length, breadth, elevation (above undamaged skin surface), and depth of infiltration into soft tissues below the skin surface and how this measurements responded to hyaluronidase injection [60]. The authors concluded that ultrasound evaluation was feasible and might offer a way to provide a more detailed and objective assessment of PIVIE tissue injury. However, further work and refinement was required to develop standardised protocols before it could become a practical tool [60].

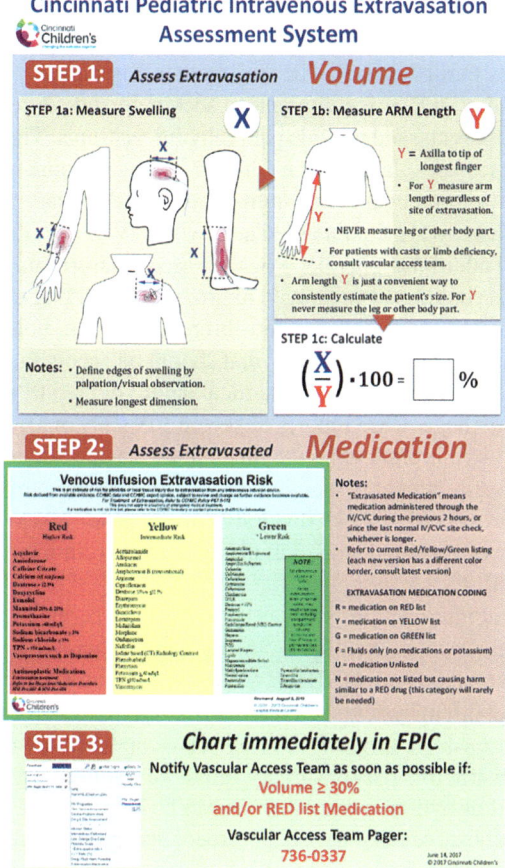

Fig. 5.4 The Cincinnati Children's Hospital approach to PIVIE assessment. (Image source: Cincinnati Children's Hospital, reproduced with permission)

5.7.3   Treating PIVIE

Beyond stopping the infusion, there is little agreement between different clinical guidelines and treatment algorithms as to the exact first aid management. This situation partly reflects the lack of robust evidence available to direct decision-making and practice interventions [61, 62]. Consequently, guidelines are often based on limited evidence, theoretical reasoning, and clinical experience. For example, some guidelines advise immediate removal of the PVAD, limb elevation, and the application of warm or cool compress. Others recommend initially retaining the PVAD in place to enable aspiration of the infiltrated fluid or administering an appropriate pharmacological treatment [63]. The application of heat or cold is contentious, particularly in cases of extravasation [59]. Localised cooling can reduce inflammatory response but will also slow metabolism of the extravasated fluid and tissue repair. Conversely, whilst warmth can enable swifter fluid dispersion, it might also increase tissue injury [59]. In the absence of definitive guidance, healthcare providers should adhere to local guidelines regarding limb elevation or the application of warm or cool compresses as part of their PIVIE management strategy.

During initial 'first aid', it is important to seek help and advice at an early time, inform the infant's parents, and provide pain reliving measures. The repertoire of non-pharmacological measures described in Chap. 4 is largely applicable. However, it is important for nurses to recognise that unlike the procedural pain experience associated with PVAD insertion, the pain associated with PIVIE can often be more severe and prolonged and additional pharmacological based measures might be appropriate. Regardless, parents should be encouraged to provide comforting touch. If parents are absent, then healthcare providers' comfort through touching, holding, and cuddling can help reduce pain and stress responses and should be encouraged [64].

Treatment depends upon the exact chemical nature of the infiltrated fluid and the severity of tissue damage. Case reports of severe PIVIE being treated using subcutaneously injected hyaluronidase/saline mixes into the site suggest positive results [7, 49, 57, 65]. This treatment is thought to work by the action of the enzyme hyaluronidase, which reversibly breaks down hyaluronic acid (a key component of the extracellular matrix) to facilitate quicker dispersion and dilution of the extravasated fluid [7, 63, 66–68].

Pharmacological interventions such as topical 2% glycerine trinitrate or subcutaneous phentolamine can be helpful counteracting the vasoconstrictive effects of vasoactive infiltrated medications. However, if used the infant needs to be carefully monitored for inadvertent systemic effects such as hypotension or reflex tachycardia [63, 66–68]. In rare cases, surgical wash out or wound debridement and later skin grafting and reconstructive plastic surgery might be required [69]. Wound dressing using hydrocolloid or hydrogel formulations can be helpful [70]. Chan et al. [68] in a single unit study observed that targeted protocol driven education to increase nurse knowledge and their compliance with PIVIE preventative care bundles can reduce the incidence of PIVIE. Despite the lack of definitive evidence concerning optimal treatment of PIVIE guidance based on current knowledge, patient and unit contextual factors and practice based experience can help prevent further patient injury. Figure 5.5 outlines one approach for developing a treatment plan for PIVIE based on first principles and current ideas about best practices (Text Boxes 5.3, 5.4 and 5.5).

Text Box 5.3 Practice Points: Things to Do
Ensuring Safe Therapy
- Use infusion devices capable of accurately delivering low infusion volumes and configured for use in this patient group.
- Implement a system of frequent and routine inspection for complications.
- For example, hourly nurse-led TLC assessment combined with parental observations together with continuous site monitoring with optical sensor technology can lead to earlier notification and reduced severity.
- Remove the PVAD when it is no longer required for therapy, complications occur, or if changes in therapy would be better delivered by other options.

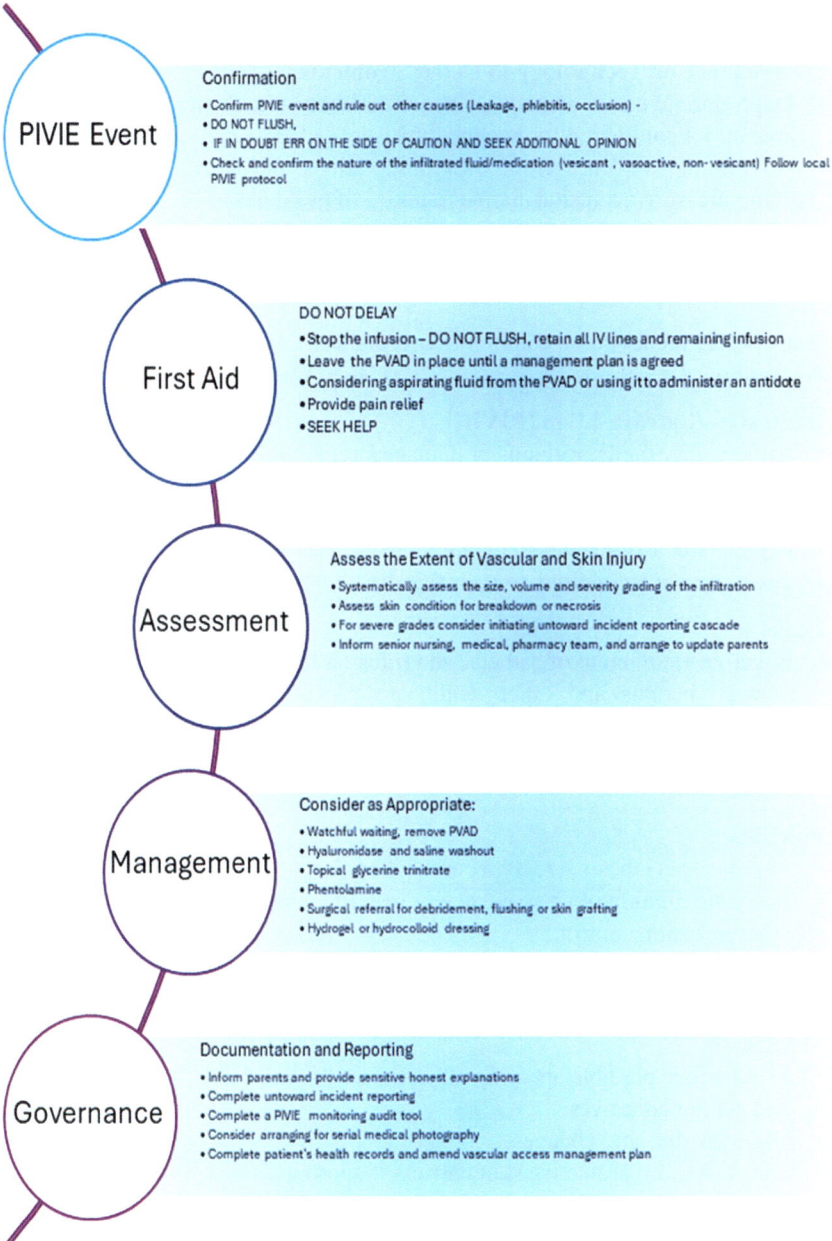

Confirmation

- Confirm PIVIE event and rule out other causes (Leakage, phlebitis, occlusion) -
- DO NOT FLUSH,
- IF IN DOUBT ERR ON THE SIDE OF CAUTION AND SEEK ADDITIONAL OPINION
- Check and confirm the nature of the infiltrated fluid/medication (vesicant , vasoactive, non-vesicant) Follow local PIVIE protocol

DO NOT DELAY

- Stop the infusion – DO NOT FLUSH, retain all IV lines and remaining infusion
- Leave the PVAD in place until a management plan is agreed
- Considering aspirating fluid from the PVAD or using it to administer an antidote
- Provide pain relief
- SEEK HELP

Assess the Extent of Vascular and Skin Injury

- Systematically assess the size, volume and severity grading of the infiltration
- Assess skin condition for breakdown or necrosis
- For severe grades consider initiating untoward incident reporting cascade
- Inform senior nursing, medical, pharmacy team, and arrange to update parents

Consider as Appropriate:

- Watchful waiting, remove PVAD
- Hyaluronidase and saline washout
- Topical glycerine trinitrate
- Phentolamine
- Surgical referral for debridement, flushing or skin grafting
- Hydrogel or hydrocolloid dressing

Documentation and Reporting

- Inform parents and provide sensitive honest explanations
- Complete untoward incident reporting
- Complete a PIVIE monitoring audit tool
- Consider arranging for serial medical photography
- Complete patient's health records and amend vascular access management plan

Fig. 5.5 A possible schematic for treating PIVIE

Text Box 5.4 Practice Points: Mistakes to Avoid

Overreliance on Technology to Detect Problems

- Inappropriate use of technology acquired from other clinical areas unsuitable or not configured for neonatal use.
- Discounting evidence from own observations and trusting on infusion pump pressure/occlusion alarms to notify of problems.

Text Box 5.5 Practice Point: Commonly Encountered Complications and Their Prevention

Infiltration/Extravasation (PIVIE)

- Avoid using fragile, tortuous or damaged veins for PVAD insertion.
- Use vein visualisation technologies for insertion.
- Proper catheter securement.
- Regular site assessments (TLC method)—educate parents in use.
- Use of sensor technology (e.g., ivWatch).

Leaks

- Effective securement of catheter and infusion lines.
- Educate parents and other healthcare providers on correct handling techniques.
- Ensure infant comfort and pain relief.
- Protect sleep.

Phlebitis

- Appropriate catheter size, type, and material.
- Adequate dilution of or avoidance of irritating medications.
- Strict infection control.
- Proper catheter securement and insertion site sealing using cyanoacrylate tissue adhesive.

MARSI

- Avoid where possible applying adhesives to the skin.
- Use gentler adhesives.
- Minimise dressing changes.
- Consider using protective skin barriers if appropriate.
- Careful application and removal of tapes and adhesives.

5.8 Concluding Remarks

This chapter has considered complications occurring during peripheral vascular access and infusion therapy. Despite improvements in practice, materials science and manufacturing PVADs continue to be the single biggest cause of iatrogenic harm in NICUs. In part, this is due to innate characteristics of sick and preterm infants, but a large element can be attributed to factors within the control of nurses and other healthcare providers. Correct use of smart infusion pump systems can improve infusion safety. Integrating nurse-led intermittent patient observation of catheter insertion sites with continuous monitoring technologies can help with earlier notification of PIVIE events and reduce their severity. Parents, when prepared and supported to do so can play an important and influential role in observing their infants for the onset of complications and providing comfort and pain relief should they occur. The treatment of complications is challenging, and the evidence-base is underdeveloped. However, some healthcare technologies including optical sensors show promise in earlier notification of complications reducing their severity.

Key Points
- n-SPC use is associated with a range of potential complications that are frequent in occurrence and problematical in terms of infant well-being and outcomes.
  - Nurses need to be proactive in their practices and vigilant in their observations to prevent these complications.
  - Parents who are made aware of what to observe for are able to better advocate for their infant and add an additional layer of protection.
- Smart infusion pump systems, when used correctly by knowledgably users can improve patient safety.
- Considerable efforts are being made in the field of neonatal vascular access to prevent or obtain earlier notification of problems and limit the severity of complications, particularly around PIVIE, mechanical phlebitis, and MARSI.
- PVAD complications like MARSI and PIVIE are painful and invariably stressful.
  - Using non-pharmacological pain relief and comfort measures is essential.
  - Their use can help to demonstrate how ethical and compassionate care principles are applied in practice.
- PIVIE is a potentially serious and life-altering complication.
  - Robust empirical evidence concerning the efficacy of different treatment regimens is underdeveloped and requires further study.
- TLC integrated with real-time sensor-based technologies can aid earlier detection of complications and reduce their severity.
- Preventing complications is better for patient well-being.
- Careful pre-procedural vascular assessment, matching of device and route to the intended fluid characteristics and therapy duration, combined with careful insertion, securement, and protection of the insertion site by dressing.

Reflective Activity

Read the following case related to a complication arising from vascular access and consider your responses to the reflective questions at the end.

> Freya, an active term born infant, now 2 days old was admitted to the NICU from the inpatient postnatal for a short course of intravenous antibiotics for suspected sepsis. She has n-SPC located in her left ankle with a continuous fluid infusion delivered by an infusion pump. Freya's parents are keen to establish breastfeeding and seem confident in lifting her from her cot to do this. The infusion pump intermittently alarms 'occlusion' about six times every hour. On examination, there are no untoward signs, and the problem is thought due to positioning of the n-SPC as repositioning the limb relieves the pressure. The alarms have become so frequent that Freya's parents note that nurses automatically silence the alarm. On shift handover, you see that the n-SPC has become dislodged, and fluid is leaking into the dressing. Freya's parents express concern and considerable annoyance at this development.

Considering the above case and your reading in this chapter, reflect on your answers to the following questions:

1. How would you respond to Freya's parents' concerns and how will you resolve their grievance?
   (a) Consider the need for honest and open communication and how you might build more trustful relationships.
   (b) Think about the legitimacy of their concerns and how staff behaviours in this case might have communicated an apparent careless attitude towards responding the equipment alarms.
2. What could have been done differently to reduce the likelihood of this situation developing?
   (a) Think, given Freya's gestational age and activity was this the optimal site? Could the n-SPC have been better secured? Were infusion pump alarm parameters set correctly? How was the actual management of these alarms conveyed to her parents? Were Freya's parents instructed on how to hold and handle her to avoid the risk of catheter dislodgment?
3. What would be the nature of your feedback to your colleague and shift lead?
   (a) Consider what would be the key points you wished to convey?
   (b) What would you document and where?

References

1. van Rens MFPT, Bayoumi MA, van de Hoogen A, Francia ALV, Cabanillas IJ, van Loon FHJ, et al. The ABBA project (assess better before access): a retrospective, cross-sectional study of neonatal intravascular device outcomes. Front Pediatr. 2022;10:10.980725. https://doi.org/10.3389/fped.2022.980725.

2. Legemaat M, Carr PJ, van Rens MFPT, Van Dijk M, Poslawsky IE, van den Hoogen A. Peripheral intravenous cannulation: complication rates in the neonatal population: a multicenter observational study. J Vasc Access. 2016;17(4):360–5. https://doi.org/10.5301/jva.5000558.

3. Indarwati F, Mathew S, Munday J, Keogh S. Incidence of peripheral intravenous catheter failure and complications in paediatric patients: systematic review and meta-analysis. Int J Nurs Stud. 2020;102:103488. https://doi.org/10.1016/J.IJNURSTU.2019.103488.

4. Unbeck M, Förberg U, Ygge B-M, Ehrenberg A, Petzold M, Johansson E. Peripheral venous catheter related complications are common among paediatric and neonatal patients. Acta Paediatr. 2015;104(6):566–74. https://doi.org/10.1111/apa.12963.

5. de Oliveira MJ, Santos AS, Oliveira AJF, Costa ACL, Regne GRS, da Trindade RE, et al. Medical adhesive-related skin injuries in the neonatology department of a teaching hospital. Nurs Crit Care. 2022;27(4):583–8. https://doi.org/10.1111/nicc.12621.

6. Fumarola S, Allaway R, Callaghan R, Collier M, Downie F, Geraghty J, et al. Overlooked and underestimated: medical adhesive-related skin injuries. J Wound Care. 2020;29(Suppl 3c):S1–24. https://doi.org/10.12968/jowc.2020.29.sup3c.S1.

7. Nickel B, Gorski L, Kleidon T, Kyes A, DeVries M, Keogh S, et al. Infusion therapy standards of practice. 9th ed. J Inf Nurs. 2024;47(1S):S1–285. https://doi.org/10.1097/NAN.0000000000000532.

8. van Rens MFPT, Hugill K, Mahmah MA, Bayoumi M, Francia ALV, Garcia KLP, et al. Evaluation of unmodifiable and potentially modifiable factors affecting peripheral intravenous device-related complications in neonates: a retrospective observational study. BMJ Open. 2021;11(9):e047788. https://doi.org/10.1136/bmjopen-2020-047788.

9. van Rens MFPT, Vijlbrief D, Braun S, Hugill K, van Loon FHJ, van de Hoogen A. Peripheral intravenous therapy infiltration/extravasation (PIVIE) risks and the potential for earlier notification of events using a novel sensor technology in a neonatal population. J Vasc Access. 2023;25:1801. https://doi.org/10.1177/11297298231185536.

10. Mannan K, Chow P, Lissauer T, Godambe S. Mistaken identity of skin cleansing solution leading to extensive chemical burns in an extremely preterm infant. Acta Paediatr. 2007;96(10):1536–7. https://doi.org/10.1111/j.1651-2227.2007.00376.x.

11. Lashkari HP, Chow P, Godambe S. Aqueous 2% chlorhexidine-induced chemical burns in an extremely premature infant. Arch Dis Child Fetal Neonat Ed. 2012;97(1):F64. https://doi.org/10.1136/adc.2011.215145.

12. Lakshmanan A, Agni M, Lieu T, Fleegler E, Kipke M, Friedlich PS, et al. The impact of preterm birth <37 weeks on parents and families: a cross-sectional study in the 2 years after discharge from the neonatal intensive care unit. Health Qual of Life Outcomes. 2017;15(1):38. https://doi.org/10.1186/s12955-017-0602-3.

13. Gallagher K, Shaw C, Aladangady N, Marlow N. Parental experience of interaction with healthcare professionals during their infant's stay in the neonatal intensive care unit. Arch Dis Child Fetal Neonat Ed. 2018;103(4):F343–8. https://doi.org/10.1136/archdischild-2016-312278.

14. Voulgaridou A, Paliouras D, Deftereos S, Skarentzos K, Tsergoula E, Miltsakaki I, et al. Hospitalization in neonatal intensive care unit: parental anxiety and satisfaction. Pan Afr Med J. 2023;44:55. https://doi.org/10.11604/pamj.2023.44.55.34344.

15. Kim UR, Peterfreund RA, Lovich MA. Drug infusion systems: technologies, performance, and pitfalls. Anesth Analg. 2017;124(5):1493–505. https://doi.org/10.1213/ANE.0000000000001707.

16. van der Eijk AC, van Rens RM, Dankelman J, Smit BJ. A literature review on flow-rate variability in neonatal IV therapy. Paediatr Anaesth. 2013;23(1):9–21. https://doi.org/10.1111/pan.12039.

17. Snijder RA, Egberts TC, Lucas P, Lemmers PM, van Bel F, Timmerman AM. Dosing errors in preterm neonates due to flow rate variability in multi-infusion syringe pump setups: an in vitro spectrophotometry study. Eur J Pharmaceut Sci. 2016;93:56–63. https://doi.org/10.1016/j.ejps.2016.07.019.

18. Blancher M, Repellin M, Maignan M, Clapé C, Perrin A, Labarère J, et al. Accuracy of low-weight versus standard syringe infusion pump devices depending on altitude. Scand J Trauma, Resus Emerg Med. 2019;27 https://doi.org/10.1186/s13049-019-0643-1.
19. Krysiak K, Cleary B, McCallion N, O'Brien F. The effect of patient's body weight, infusion connection point, and infusion pump position on intravenous multi-infusion drug delivery at low infusion rates suitable for premature neonates. J Pharm Pharmacol. 2023;76:34–43. https://doi.org/10.1093/jpp/rgad108.
20. Jonckers T, Berger I, Kuijten T, Meijer E, Andriessen P. The effect of in-line infusion filtering on in-line pressure monitoring in an experimental infusion system for newborns. Neonat Netw. 2014;33(3):133–7.
21. Chua J, Ratnavadivel A. Comparison of flow pressures in different 3-way infusion devices: an in-vitro study. Patient Saf Surg. 2018;12:19. https://doi.org/10.1186/s13037-018-0165-1.
22. Oh EJ, Hong KY, Lee JH, Kim DK, Cho J, Min JJ. Simulation analysis of flow rate variability during microinfusions: the effect of vertical displacement and multidrug infusion in conventional infusion pumps versus new cylinder-type infusion pumps. Anesth Analg. 2022;134(1):59–68. https://doi.org/10.1213/ANE.0000000000005736.
23. van der Eijk AC, van der Plas AJ, van der Palen CJ, Dankelman J, Smit BJ. In vitro measurement of flow rate variability in neonatal IV therapy with and without the use of check valves. J Neonat Perinat Med. 2014;7(1):55–64. https://doi.org/10.3233/NPM-1475213.
24. Snijder RA, Konings MK, Lucas P, Egberts TC, Timmerman AD. Flow variability and its physical causes in infusion technology: a systematic review of in vitro measurement and modelling studies. Biomed Tech (Berl). 2015;60(4):277–300. https://doi.org/10.1515/bmt-2014-0148.
25. Rathore N, Pranay P, Eu B, Ji W, Walls E. Variability in syringe components and its impact on functionality of delivery systems. PDA J Pharm Sci Technol. 2011;65(5):468–80. https://doi.org/10.5731/pdajpst.2011.00785.
26. Baeckert M, Batliner M, Grass B, Buehler PK, Daners MS, Meboldt M, et al. Performance of modern syringe infusion pump assemblies at low infusion rates in the perioperative setting. Br J Anaesth. 2020;124(2):173–82. https://doi.org/10.1016/j.bja.2019.10.007.
27. Schmidt N, Saez C, Seri I, Maturana A. Impact of syringe size on the performance of infusion pumps at low flow rates. Pediatr Crit Care Med. 2010;11(2):282–6. https://doi.org/10.1097/PCC.0b013e3181c31848.
28. Tooke LJ, Howell L. Syringe drivers: incorrect selection of syringe type from the syringe menu may result in significant errors in drug delivery. Anaesth Intensive Care. 2014;42(4):467–72. https://doi.org/10.1177/0310057X1404200407.
29. Bergon-Sendin E, Perez-Grande C, Lora-Pablos D, Moral-Pumarega MT, Melgar-Bonis A, Peña-Peloche C, et al. Smart pumps and random safety audits in a neonatal intensive care unit: a new challenge for patient safety. BMC Pediatr. 2015;15:206. https://doi.org/10.1186/s12887-015-0521-6.
30. Melton KR, Timmons K, Walsh KE, Meinzen-Derr JK, Kirkendall E. Smart pumps improve medication safety but increase alert burden in neonatal care. BMC Med Informatics Decision Making. 2019;19:213. https://doi.org/10.1186/s12911-019-0945-2.
31. Schnock KO, Rostas SE, Yoon CS, Lipsitz S, Bates DW, Dykes PC. Intravenous medication administration safety with smart infusion pumps in the neonatal intensive care unit: an observational study. Drug Saf. 2024;47(1):29–38. https://doi.org/10.1007/s40264-023-01365-6.
32. Waterson J, Bedner A. Types and frequency of infusion pump alarms and infusion-interruption to infusion-recovery times for critical short half-life infusions: retrospective data analysis. JMIR. Hum Factors. 2019;6(3):e14123. https://doi.org/10.2196/14123.
33. Sendelbach S, Funk M. Alarm fatigue: a patient safety concern. AACN Adv Crit Care. 2013;24(4):378–86. https://doi.org/10.1097/NCI.0b013e3182a903f9.
34. Lewandowska K, Weisbrot M, Cieloszyk A, Mędrzycka-Dąbrowska W, Krupa S, Ozga D. Impact of alarm fatigue on the work of nurses in an intensive care environment-a systematic review. Int J Environ Res Public Health. 2020;17(22):8409. https://doi.org/10.3390/ijerph17228409.

35. Dee SA, Tucciarone J, Plotkin G, Mallilo C. Determining the impact of an alarm management program on alarm fatigue among ICU and telemetry RNs: an evidence based research project. SAGE Open Nurs. 2022;8 https://doi.org/10.1177/23779608221098713.

36. Gündoğan G, Erdağı OS. The effects of alarm fatigue on the tendency to make medical errors in nurses working in intensive care units. Nurs Crit Care. 2023;28(6):996–1003. https://doi.org/10.1111/nicc.12969.

37. de Azevedo Bringel JM, Abreu I, Muniz M-CMC, de Almeida PC, Silva M-GG. Excessive noise in neonatal units and the occupational stress experienced by healthcare professionals: an assessment of burnout and measurement of cortisol levels. Healthcare. 2023;11(14):2002. https://doi.org/10.3390/healthcare11142002.

38. Albanowski K, Burdick KJ, Bonafide CP, Kleinpell R, Schlesinger JJ. Ten years later, alarm fatigue is still a safety concern. AACN Adv Crit Care. 2023;34(3):189–97. https://doi.org/10.4037/aacnacc2023662. PMID: 37644627

39. Joint Commission International (JCI). JCI accreditation standards for hospitals. 7th ed. Oakbrook Terrace: JCI; 2020.

40. Gouveia SM. In-line pressure monitoring in IV infusions: benefits for patients and nurses. Br J Nurs. 2016;25(19):S28–33. https://doi.org/10.12968/bjon.2016.25.19.S28.

41. Friedman J, Friedman SH, Collin M, Martin RJ. Staff perceptions of challenging parent-staff interactions and beneficial strategies in the neonatal intensive care unit. Acta Paediatr. 2018;107(1):33–9. https://doi.org/10.1111/apa.14025.

42. Sakonidou S, Kotzamanis S, Tallett A, Poots AJ, Modi N, Bell D, et al. Parents' experiences of communication in neonatal care (PEC): a neonatal survey refined for real-time parent feedback. Arch Dis Child Fetal Neonat Ed. 2023;108(4):F416–20. https://doi.org/10.1136/archdischild-2022-324548.

43. Danski MT, Mingorance P, Johann DA, Vayego SA, Lind J. Incidência de complicações locais e fatores de risco associados ao cateter intravenoso periférico em neonates [Incidence of local complications and risk factors associated with peripheral intravenous catheter in neonates]. Rev Esc Enferm USP. 2016;50(1):22–8. https://doi.org/10.1590/S0080-623420160000100003.

44. Baye ND, Teshome AA, Ayenew AA, Amare TJ, Mulu AT, Abebe EC, et al. Incidence, time to occurrence and predictors of peripheral intravenous cannula -related complications among neonates and infants in Northwest Ethiopia: an institutional-based prospective study. BMC Nurs. 2023;22:11. https://doi.org/10.1186/s12912-022-01164-x.

45. Pettit J. Assessment of the infant with a peripheral intravenous device. Adv Neonat Care. 2003;3(5):230–40. https://doi.org/10.1053/s1536-0903(03)00171-1.

46. McNichol L, Lund C, Rosen T, Gray M. Medical adhesives and patient safety: state of the science: consensus statements for the assessment, prevention, and treatment of adhesive-related skin injuries. J Wound Ostomy Continence Nurs. 2013;40(4):365–80. https://doi.org/10.1097/WON.0b013e3182995516.

47. ivWatch LLC. ivWatch® breakthrough in IV safety, whitepaper. 2023. ivWatch-Model-400-Whitepaper.pdf. Accessed 12 August 2024.

48. Doellman D, Rineair S. The use of optical detection for continuous monitoring of pediatric IV sites. JAVA. 2019;24(2):44–7. https://doi.org/10.2309/j.java.2019.002.003.

49. Yew CK, Mat Johar SFN, Lim WY. Case series of neonatal extravasation injury: importance of early identification and management. Cureus. 2022;14(1):e21179. https://doi.org/10.7759/cureus.21179.

50. Graham YP, Heim C, Goodman SH, Miller AH, Nemeroff CB. The effects of neonatal stress on brain development: implications for psychopathology. Dev Psychopathol. 1999;11(3):545–65. https://doi.org/10.1017/s0954579499002205.

51. Smith GC, Gutovich J, Smyser C, Pineda R, Newnham C, Tjoeng TH, et al. Neonatal intensive care unit stress is associated with brain development in preterm infants. Ann Neurol. 2011;70(4):541–9. https://doi.org/10.1002/ana.22545.

52. Vinall J, Miller SP, Bjornson BH, Fitzpatrick KPV, Poskitt KJ, Brant R, et al. Invasive procedures in preterm children: brain and cognitive development at school age. Pediatr. 2014;133(3):412–21. https://doi.org/10.1542/peds.2013-1863.

53. Lund C. Medical adhesives in the NICU. Newborn Inf Nurs Rev. 2014;14(4):160–5.
54. van Rens MFPT, Spencer TR, Hugill K, Francia AL, van Loon FHJ, Bayoumi MA. Octyl-butyl-cyanoacrylate glue for securement of peripheral intravenous catheters: a retrospective observational study in the neonatal population. J Vasc Access. 2023;16:11297298231154629. https://doi.org/10.1177/11297298231154629.
55. Cincinnati paediatric intravenous extravasation assessment system. 2017. http://cincinnatichildrens.org/service/v/vascular-access/hcp. Accessed 12 August 2024.
56. D'Andrea V, Prontera G, Carlino R, Di Trani H, Carlettini I, Pittiruti M, et al. Optical detection of infiltration during peripheral intravenous infusion in neonates. J Vasc Access. 2023;25:1780. https://doi.org/10.1177/11297298231177723.
57. Dufficy M, Takashima M, Cunninghame J, Griffin BR, McBride CA, August D, et al. Extravasation injury management for neonates and children: a systematic review and aggregated case series. J Hosp Med. 2022;17(10):832–42. https://doi.org/10.1002/jhm.12951.
58. National Infusion and Vascular Access Society, (NIVAS). NIVAS infiltration and extravasation toolkit. https://vascularaccess.files/svdcdn.com/production/images/NIVAS-Infiltration-and-Extravasation-toolkit-version-1-Feb-2024b.pdf?dm=1734439180. Accessed 12 Jan 2025.
59. Tofani B, Rineair S, Gosdin CH, Pilcher PM, McGee S, Varadarajan KR, et al. Quality improvement project to reduce infiltration and extravasation events in a pediatric hospital. J Pediatr Nurs. 2012;27(6):682–9. https://doi.org/10.1016/j.pedn.2012.01.005.
60. Boyar V, Galiczewski C, Kurepa D. Point- of-care ultrasound use in neonatal peripheral intravenous extravasation injuries. J Wound care Ostomy Continence Nurs. 2018;45(6):503–9. https://doi.org/10.1097/WON.0000000000000475.
61. Corbett M, Marshall D, Harden M, Oddie S, Phillips R, McGuire W. Treating extravasation injuries in infants and young children: a scoping review and survey of UK NHS practice. BMC Pediatr. 2019;19(1):6. https://doi.org/10.1186/s12887-018-1387-13061.
62. Baird J, Lindstadt K, Wu UC. A call to action: establishing an evidence base for pediatric extravasation injury management. J Hosp Med. 2022;17(12):1033–4. https://doi.org/10.1002/jhm.12965.
63. Hackenberg RK, Kabir K, Müller A, Heydweiller A, Burger C, Welle K. Extravasation injuries of the limbs in neonates and children—development of a treatment algorithm. Dtsch Arztebl Int. 2021;118(33–34):547–54. https://doi.org/10.3238/arztebl.m2021.0220.
64. Nist MD, Robinson A, Harrison TM, Pickler RH. An integrative review of clinician-administered comforting touch interventions and acute stress responses of preterm infants. J Pediatr Nurs. 2022;67:e113–22. https://doi.org/10.1016/j.pedn.2022.08.020.
65. van Rens MFPT, Hugill K, Francia ALV, Abdelwahab AH, Garcia KLO. Treatment of a neonatal peripheral intravenous infiltration/extravasation (PIVIE) injury with hyaluronidase: a case report. JAVA. 2021;26(4):32–7. https://doi.org/10.2309/JAVA-D-21-00010. Reprinted in Br J Nurs. 2022;31(8):S31-6. https://doi.org/10.12968/bjon.2022.31.8.S31
66. Beall V, Hall B, Mulholland JT, Gephart SM. Neonatal extravasation: an overview and algorithm for evidence-based treatment. Newborn Infant Nurs Rev. 2013;13(4):189–95. https://doi.org/10.1053/j.nainr.2013.09.001.
67. Gopalakrishnan PN, Goel N, Banerjee S. Saline irrigation for the management of skin extravasation injury in neonates. Cochrane Database Syst Rev. 2017;7(7):CD008404. https://doi.org/10.1002/14651858.CD008404.pub3.
68. Chan KM, Chau JPC, Choi KC, et al. Clinical practice guideline on the prevention and management of neonatal extravasation injury: a before-and-after study design. BMC Pediatr. 2020;20:445. https://doi.org/10.1186/s12887-020-02346-9.
69. Maruccia M, Tedeschi P, Corrao C, Elia R, La Padula S, Di Summa PG, et al. Meek micro-skin grafting and acellular dermal matrix in pediatric patients: a novel approach to massive extravasation injury. J Clin Med. 2023;12(14):4587. https://doi.org/10.3390/jcm12144587.
70. Steen EH, Wang X, Boochoon KS, Ewing DC, Strang HE, et al. Wound healing and wound care in neonates: current therapies and novel options. Adv Skin Wound Care. 2020;33(6):294–300. https://doi.org/10.1097/01.ASW.0000661804.09496.8c.

Central Vascular Access Devices

6

Chapter Learning Objectives

Upon completing this chapter, readers will be able to:

- Differentiate the various types of central vascular access devices (CVADs) used in neonatal care settings by their design, insertion technique, and suitability for particular therapies.
  - Specifically: n-PICC/ECC, CICC and FICC (tunnelled and non-tunnelled).
- Critically evaluate CVAD insertion techniques.
  - With a focus on the modified Seldinger technique (MST) and infection, to make informed decisions about the most appropriate insertion technique.
- Advocate for effective comfort promotion and pain-relieving strategies during CVAD insertion.
- Apply knowledge of CVAD-related complications to develop preventative strategies and implement management plans should complications occur.
- Critically reflect on the pivotal role of parents in contributing to the safety and well-being of their infant with a CVAD.

6.1 Introduction

Central vascular access devices (CVADs) are frequently used for delivering vascular therapies and monitoring vital signs in neonatal intensive care units (NICU). Together they form a clinically important group of devices that complements short and long peripheral catheters (n-SPC, n-LPC) options explored in Chapters 4 and 5. CVADs are available in several different materials and designs for specific uses (see Chap. 3 for an overview of catheter materials). Device subtypes (Table 6.1) include neonatal-peripherally inserted central catheters (n-PICCs), also known as epicutaneo-caval catheters (ECCs). These terms have been introduced to ensure greater clarity and substitute for less precise terms such as 'long line', 'percutaneous central line', and

M. R. van Rens, K. Hugill, *Vascular Access in Neonatal Nursing Practice: A Neuroprotective Approach*, https://doi.org/10.1007/978-3-031-81602-4_6

Table 6.1   The range of central vascular catheters for neonatal use

Type of device	Insertion method	Ultrasound guidance	Typical dwell time[a]
Umbilical venous catheter (UVC)[b]	Direct insertion	Possible	<5 days
Femoral inserted central catheter (FICC) Non-tunnelled and tunnelled	Modified Seldinger technique (MST)	Essential	>14 days
Central inserted central catheter (CICC) Non-tunnelled and tunnelled	MST	Essential	>14 days
Neonatal-peripherally inserted central catheter (n-PICC)/epicutaneo-caval catheter (ECC)	MST Steel split needle Peelable cannula Fine-tipped	Desirable	>7 to <14 days

[a]Dwell times can vary based on clinical need and local risk assessment
[b]See Chap. 7

'PICC' [1, 2]. Femorally inserted central catheters (FICC) and centrally inserted central catheters (CICCs) were once seldom seen outside of specialist centres. Now these devices, in their non-tunnelled and tunnelled versions are being regularly integrated into NICU practice. Umbilical catheters are often placed in the central vasculature of recently born infants and therefore should be considered as a specialist variety of CVAD used in this patient group. The insertion, use, range of specific complications, and their prevention and management are considered in the next chapter.

This chapter places emphasis on n-PICC/ECC insertion and management to provide structure and consideration of issues that have a wider impact on CVAD use. This focus reflects many nurses' greater familiarity with these devices and area of practice in which nurses have become increasingly involved as lead practitioners (Text Box 6.1).

Text Box 6.1 Practice Point: n-PICC/ECC and Adult/Paediatric PICC
n-PICC/ECCs as used with infants are fundamentally dissimilar from PICCs used with children and adults [1].
   n-PICC/ECCs are:

- Generally, 1–2 Fr
- Usually made of polyurethane (PUR) and less frequently silicone
- Usually inserted via superficial veins of the limbs or scalp using direct vein visualisation technology or ultrasound guidance

PICCs as used in paediatrics and adults are:

- Often 3 Fr and more
- Often made of new-generation PURs, making them power-injectable
- Frequently inserted directly into the deep veins of the arm (brachial, basilic, axillary) using ultrasound guidance

(continued)

> **Text Box 6.1** (continued)
>
> These differences translate into different performances, PICCs are suitable for:
>
> - Blood sampling
> - High flow infusion (up to 1 mL/second versus 1 mL/minute for n-PICC/ECC)
> - Hemodynamic monitoring
> - Infusing blood products
> - Extended dwell times, up to many months
>
> Performances more akin to CICC or FICC are seen in neonates.

6.2   Selecting the Most Appropriate CVAD

The design and configuration of different CVAD catheters is tailored for their intended therapeutic use, vascular route, and insertion technique. These attributes confer specific advantages, limitations, complication risks, and indicate when their use is appropriate [3–6]. All CVADs can be used to infuse fluids that are incompatible with peripheral vein infusion. Such fluids include those which are hyperosmolar (600 mOsm/L) or have a pH <5 or >9 or carry a high risk of vascular injury. All central vascular catheters, except for those inserted through umbilical blood vessels can be used for long-term intravenous therapies [7–9]. The main time limiting factor relates to the increased likelihood of complications, including infection. The choice of CVAD is based on consideration of several factors in the neonatal vascular access management plan (n-VAMP), including:

- Patient factors
  - Size (weight), clinical situation (stable, unstable; routine, urgent, emergency), circulatory performance, systematic vascular and skin integrity assessments, preexisting morbidities, age post-birth, previous vascular access history
- Therapy factors
  - Intended duration, infusate characteristics, need for single or multiple co-infusions, flow rates required (maximum and/or minimum), haemodynamic monitoring requirements, need for frequent blood sampling
- Pragmatic factors
  - Availability of required consumables and ultrasound, education, training, and competence of healthcare providers

Consideration of these factors should be incorporated into an individualised vascular access management plan (n-VAMP), see Chap. 2.

6.2.1 N-PICC/ECC

n-PICC/ECCs single lumen polyurethane (PUR) 1 Fr n-PICC/ECCs are particularly suitable for infants weighing less than 1 K. Double lumen devices can provide an option for co-infusing incompatible fluids. Although these catheters are typically larger in size due to engineering considerations, they may be unsuitable for smaller infants [7, 10, 11]. Pre-procedural vascular assessment (visual, with or without technology and ultrasound-guided) can help determine the suitability of individual veins. Anticipated dwell times of more than 5 days can be used as guide when considering this device. When the therapy duration is anticipated to be longer than 14 days, a tunnelled or non-tunnelled CICC or FICC might be the more appropriate choice.

6.2.2 CICC and FICC

CICCs and FICCs have several advantages over other options. Catheters are available in larger sizes allowing increased flow rates, hemodynamic monitoring, and the possibility for frequent blood sampling (which can help preserve peripheral blood vessels) [12, 13]. The tunnelled versions can last several months in situ without significantly escalating infection risks. However, competence in using ultrasound is essential for guiding safe insertion. Furthermore, because of the need for precise positioning, infants need to be sedated or anesthetised which might be undesirable for some infants [3].

6.3 Selecting the Appropriate Vessel for CVAD Placement

Preterm infants have anatomically underdeveloped and fragile veins with narrower lumens compared to older patients. These features present considerable engineering challenges to manufacture clinically useable devices. Due to these constraints and a desire to reduce the likelihood of complications, it is essential to undertake systematic pre-procedural assessment of blood vessel suitability [14]. Doing this can help to ensure successful insertion, optimal catheter tip location, and reduce complications (Text Box 6.2).

Text Box 6.2 Practice Point: Choosing a CVAD or n-SPC?

A newborn infant 30 + 2 weeks gestation, weighing 1850 g, is predicted to require 7 days of intravenous parenteral nutrition.

Given this information, what is the best choice of vascular access? Consider the following factors:

- n-PICC insertion takes around 1.4 skin breaking procedure to insert
- Average n-PICC indwell-time is more than 14 days
- The complication rate after insertion for n-PICC is around 11% [5].
- n-SPC insertion takes around 2.1 skin breaking procedures to insert
- Average n-SPC dwell time is 32 h
- Complication rate after insertion for n-SPC is about 55% [5, 15].

Only 1 n-PICC would be needed for the required therapy duration using 1.4 insertion attempts. In contrast, 5.3 n-SPCs would be needed and 11 attempts are required.

The choice that results in a better infant experience is obvious.

6.3.1 Blood Vessel Suitability Assessment

Before CVAD insertion, it is essential to assess vein anatomy, calibre, and depth for suitability to accommodate the intended device, indeed:

The choice of the vein is of the utmost importance and should be obtained after a rational and objective systematic evaluation [14, p. 2].

Standardised protocols have been developed to support systematic assessment using ultrasound before catheterisation. They include:

- RaPeVA (rapid peripheral vein assessment)
- RaCeVA (rapid central vein assessment)
- RaFeVA (rapid femoral vein assessment) [14, 16–18]

The three protocols focus on different parts of the vasculature and aim to identify optimal veins for insertion. For example, RaCeVA [17] follows a series of seven steps similar in structure to the RaSuVa tool described in Chap. 5. The intent of this protocol is to use ultrasound to systematically assess the anatomy, size, and suitability of veins in the upper body and visualise adjacent tissues (nerves, for example) prior to central vascular access.

Recently, subcutaneous tunnelled CICC and FICCs have become more widely used in practice. This is due to an increasing body of evidence that supports their utility and safety in neonatal populations [12, 13, 19–21] coupled with increasing numbers of healthcare providers developing expertise in using this approach. One of the main benefits of tunnelling is separation of the venipuncture and skin exit sites. This can reduce extraluminal contamination and the chance of accidental removal. One decisional aid, the rapid assessment of vascular exit site and tunnelling options (RAVESTO) [22] seeks to methodically determine the best exit sites for a tunnelled device. The tool can be applied to neonates.

6.3.2 Catheter-to-Vein Ratio

Vein sizes vary between anatomical sites and individuals [23]. The catheter-to-vein ratio (C:V ratio) typically refers to the size relationship between the catheter and vein [24]. Using this ratio helps determine the safest catheter size for any given vein helping to avoid overly disrupting blood flow and thrombotic complications [24–27].

Sharp et al. [26] in a study of adults with a PICC and symptomatic thrombosis reported that modelling of C:V ratios exceeding 45% was predictive of thrombosis. However, this figure had wide confidence intervals and might not be readily transferable to neonatal vasculatures, so should be treated with caution. Based on simulated modelling [27], a common recommendation in neonates is to maintain a C:V ratio of 1:3 (33%) [3, 7]. This means that a catheter should ideally not occupy more than 1/3 (33%) of the blood vessel lumen. Figure 6.1 graphically illustrates

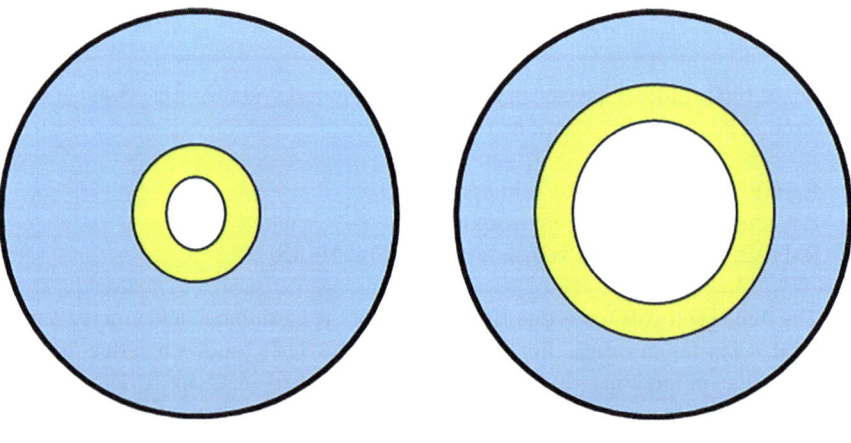

Catheter:Vein ratio approximately 33%   Catheter:Vein ratio approximately 60%
1 Fr catheter in a 1 mm diameter vein   2 Fr catheter in a 1 mm diameter vein

Blood vessel lumen in blue
Catheter wall yellow and lumen in white

Fig. 6.1 Visualising catheter-to-vein ratios

this relationship. In practice, a 1 Fr catheter would ideally be inserted into a vein of 1 mm or more diameter. A 2 Fr catheter would require a 2 mm diameter vein to maintain this ratio (see Sect. 6.3.3), but locating a vein of this size in the extremely preterm infant can be challenging. Web-based applications are available to calculate this ratio, a useful example is 'CVR Calc 2.0' (https://vascularaccess.com.au/catheter-vessel-ratio/).

In practice, C:V ratio provides general guidance. Healthcare providers may consider various other factors (see Sect. 6.2) when deciding on catheter size.

6.3.3   Catheter Sizing

There are two main systems to describe the size of vascular devices: Gauge and French. French gauge, variously abbreviated as Fr, FR, or F was devised to measure the outer diameter of surgical catheters. According to some sources, it is called the 'Charriere Gauge' (CH or Ch) in honour of its inventor [28]. Essentially, to determine the outer diameter in millimetre, divide the Fr size by 3. Using this formula, a 1 Fr catheter has a diameter of around 0.33 mm and a 2 Fr 0.66 mm.

The Gauge scale (abbreviated G) originated from the 'Birmingham gauge' developed to standardise industrial production of steel wire and was only later appropriated for medical use [29]. In contrast to the Fr system, G uses British imperial measurements (inch, foot, etc.) and is non-linear and inversely proportional. As G increases, the outer diameter diminishes. In practice, a 24 G needle is smaller than an 18 G. Though not directly convertible and subject to rounding errors, 28 G approximates to 1.1 Fr, 26 G to 1.4 Fr, and 24 G to 1.79 Fr.

Importantly G and Fr sizing's only reflect the outer diameter. Manufacturing processes, the inclusion of additional components, coating materials, and the number of lumens will affect internal dimensions. Manufacturers provide detailed information about the design characteristics of their products in their technical and promotional materials. This information should be consulted by users to ensure that devices meet infant needs.

6.4   CVAD Insertion

Regardless of exact technicalities, all CVAD insertion techniques emphasise similar principles. The challenges encountered by patients of all ages having central vascular catheters are similar, and their resolution requires a proactive multidisciplinary approach. The safe insertion of PICCS (SIPP) [14] and the safe insertion of central access in paediatric patients (SICA-PED) [30] protocols have many commonalties. The SICA-PED protocol sets out a series of seven steps to direct processes around the safe insertion of central vascular devices in children [30]. These are readily relatable in neonatal settings (Text Box 6.3).

Text Box 6.3 Practice Point: The SICA-PED Protocol
1. Pre-procedural systematic evaluation of blood vessel suitability using ultrasound and RaCeVa vein assessment protocol
2. Appropriate aseptic technique
3. Clear identification of the intended venipuncture site under ultrasound guidance
4. Intra-procedural confirmation of catheter tip position using ultrasound or intracavity ECG
5. Rationalised choice of catheter exit site using assessment protocols (e.g., RAVESTO)
6. Appropriate securement of the catheter using sutureless devices and cyanoacrylate glue
7. Appropriate sealing and protection of the catheter exit site using cyanoacrylate glue and transparent dressing

Combined evidence indicates that incorporating these steps into standardised guidelines and care bundles can reduce complications associated with CVAD insertion and use [14, 24, 30].

6.4.1   Reducing Infection Risk During CVAD Insertion

Standardised frameworks and care bundles for the prevention and control of hospital acquired infections (HAI) [31] and hospital onset bacteraemia and fungemia (HOB) [32] have become core aspects of practice across all healthcare settings around the world [33–40]. The aseptic non-touch technique (ANTT®) clinical practice framework is a widely endorsed approach for infection prevention and control in vascular access [36, 39]. The choice of Standard-ANTT® or Surgical-ANTT® approaches for vascular access related procedures is determined by assessing risk [39].

Risk assessment involves consideration of the environment, technical difficulties in maintaining asepsis, and protecting all 'Key-Parts' and 'Key-Sites' [39]. Inserting and using CVADs is a high-risk procedure for infection risk. This is partly because of the duration of the procedure, the number and size of 'Key-Parts, and infants' immature immune systems. Consequently, in NICU settings, a Surgical-ANTT® approach is the most appropriate choice for CVAD insertion and dressing changes, and when removal is complex (e.g., tunnelled or damaged catheters) [39, 40].

Effective pre-procedural skin antisepsis is vital to reduce infection risk [7, 24, 31]. Most NICUs use a combination of various concentrations of chlorhexidine in aqueous or isopropyl alcohol solution, depending on local guidelines (see Chap. 4, Sect. 4.3.1). Incontrovertible evidence about the optimal choice of skin disinfection solution and routine is elusive, and further research is required. However, having a consistent systematic approach that incorporates steps to avoid chemical burns is essential.

6.4.2 CVAD Insertion Techniques

6.4.2.1 CICC and FICC

CICCs are typically inserted in the internal jugular or subclavian veins. The modified Seldinger technique (MST) and ultrasound guidance to locate the chosen vein and guide insertion are essential [12, 13, 19, 20, 41, 42]. FICC insertion follows the same technique [43]. However, with FICC tunnelling is often the preferred approach to avoid exit site contamination, accidental removal, or dislodgment [22, 24]. Unlike with n-PICC/ECCs, the independent insertion of CICCs and FICCs is generally beyond the professional scope of nurses in most NICUs. As such detailed exploration is beyond the scope of this book.

6.4.2.2 N-PICC/ECC

Traditionally, n-PICC/ECCs have been inserted using a steel splitting needle or peelable cannula technique [44, 45] into the peripheral veins of the limbs and scalp [44–46]. Whilst this technique continues to have a role in practice, it has some limitations. The needle can only accommodate 1 Fr and not larger 2 Fr catheters and there is a risk of damaging the catheter when moving the catheter through the needle or when removing and splitting the needle. Over time alternative methods have been proposed, for example, the fine-tipped [11], the Seldinger, and the MST [44, 45, 47–51]. The MST, accompanied by ultrasound has established itself as the preferred technique amongst many healthcare providers for virtually all CVAD insertions.

6.4.2.3 The Modified Seldinger Technique (MST)

The original Seldinger technique proved advantageous when inserting larger calibre catheters percutaneously. At the time, it was unique in using a flexible guidewire to direct the threading of the catheter to the central vasculature. The MST is a development of this original approach developed to mitigate some of its potential shortcomings [10, 11, 44, 48]. Figure 6.2 summarises the key steps in using the MST.

The MST involves the initial step of puncture of the selected vein with a needle cannula device, insertion of a guidewire through the needle, followed by needle removal leaving the guidewire in the vein. Next the vein is dilated, often using a bespoke aid and a catheter introducer is inserted into the vein over the guidewire. Once this step is completed, the guidewire and vein dilator are removed. Thereafter the catheter can be threaded though the introducer to its desired position, ideally under ultrasound guidance.

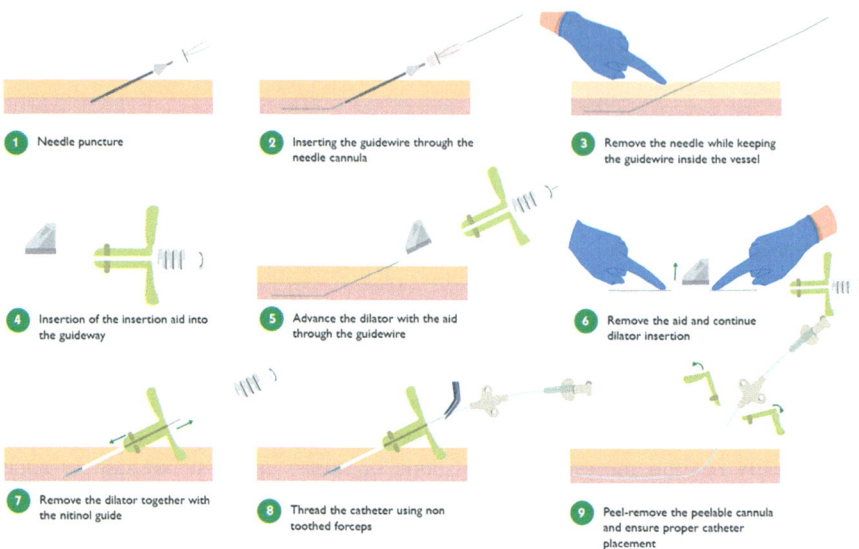

Fig. 6.2   The modified Seldinger technique (MST). (Picture courtesy of Vygon, reproduced with permission)

Preprepared kits of matched MST components suitable for neonatal use are readily available, for example, NeoMagic® (NeoMedical™), MicroSlide® (Galt™), and Microsite insertion kit: MST (Vygon). To ensure that different needles, catheters, and introducer wire combinations are matching, it can be circumspect to opt for one manufacturer's product range. Doing this will to help avoid compatibility issues that can lead to kinking, snagging, or breakage.

6.4.3   MST in n-PICC/ECC

When used for n-PICC/ECC insertion, the MST enables smaller peripheral veins to be used and can increase first-attempt and overall successful insertion rates and reduce complications associated with insertion [45, 47]. Gibb et al. [51] compared the use of the MST or the split needle technique for n-PICC/ECC insertion in preterm infants ($n = 57$). The authors reported first-attempt success of 53% for MST versus 26% for split needle ($P = 0.014$) and overall successes of 72% versus 40% ($P = 0.0046$). However, this was a single centre retrospective study with a small study population who were not randomised to the intervention or inserter.

Infants exposed to the MST were smaller, though subgroup analysis was supportive of the overall conclusions. These factors might have introduced some bias to the findings, and the results might not be generalisable.

Reports support the view that MST decreases venous trauma, and once the technique is mastered, it reduces procedure time. This in turn can contribute to reduced infant stress and handling [10, 43, 45, 52]. MST has other possible advantages. Pettit [53] outlined a technique whereby using MST it is possible to exchange the catheter mid-procedure into the same vein. This could be valuable if problems arise with the first catheter. Sometimes the course of the catheter deviates from its intended route or aligns with the blood vessel wall preventing advancement. Under ultrasound guidance withdrawing the catheter slightly, briefly pausing, and then advancing again can correct the course of the catheter [54]. Spencer [55] describes another method, the 'high-flow-flush technique'; this involves flushing the catheter to encourage the tip to align with the dominant venous blood direction (i.e., towards the direction of the heart).

Rarely guidewires encounter resistance and become difficult to remove; this situation might affect vascular integrity or failure to insert [56]. In practice, straightening and untwisting the whole length can be helpful and enable removal [44]. One novel approach uses a diluted lipid emulsion (1:9 with normal saline) as a pre-flush before insertion to overcome this potential issue [57] (Text Box 6.4).

Text Box 6.4 Practice Point: Overcoming Practical Challenges in n-PICC/ECC Insertion

- Venipuncture needles make comparatively small incisions, this can make it difficult for the vein dilator to overcome skin resistance.
  - Using an insertion angle parallel to the skin with an assistant stretching the skin and gently wriggling the dilator whilst insertion generally overcomes this problem.
- Over-rapidly advancing the catheter can lead to increased resistance and false routing.
  - Pausing and slowing advancement generally overcomes the problem (enabling the catheter to *'go with the flow'*).
- If resistance is still met, there are things might help.
  - Reposition the limb.
  - Very gently hold the catheter 'under slight pressure' for a few seconds.
  - Stretch the skin by gentle massage in the direction of flow.
  - Gently flush the catheter whilst advancing.
  - Administering a sucrose solution and providing support to help the infant reposition themselves can help reduce muscle tension.

6.4.3.1 Tip Location

n-PICC/ECC, CICC, and FICCs should have their catheter tips placed in the vena cava (inferior/superior) or around the right atrium depending on the site of insertion and performance required [3, 4, 6, 7, 10, 23]. Traditionally, catheter tip location was based on clinical assessment of the likely route, catheter length markings, experience, and a variety of predictive protocol driven calculations [58]. In many NICUs, conventual post-procedural radiology remains the main method of confirming tip position [59], it was until recently considered to be the 'gold standard'. However, this method has limitations; it is retrospective which limits opportunities to advance catheters short of their target or reposition those misrouted. Additionally, patient movement and limb positioning can affect interpretation and soft tissues are less visible. Now real-time ultrasound or IC-ECG guidance is becoming the norm during insertion and confirmation of catheter tip location [10, 27, 47, 54, 59–62]. Consequently, influential bodies [e.g., 24] state that post-procedural X-rays are not necessary if more advanced tip location technology is used.

6.5   Securement and Dressing

Choices around CVAD securement and dressing affect catheter performance and complication risks. Whilst the principles for fixation and stabilisation are generally similar (Text Box 6.5).

Text Box 6.5 Practice Point: n-PICC/ECC, CICC, FICC Securement, and Dressing

- Seal the exit site with a cyanoacrylate tissue adhesive approved for vascular access.
    - Cyanoacrylate tissue adhesive is haemostatic and bacteriostatic which reduces bleeding and kills microorganisms, thereby protecting the exit site from extraluminal contamination by microorganisms [63].
- Secure the catheter using an engineered sutureless securement device or integrated securement dressing (e.g. SecureAcath®, Interrad Medical, StatLock™, BD, Grip-Lok®, Vygon, SorbaView® Shield, Medline), or directly applied cyanoacrylate tissue adhesive on the catheter and its hub [63–67].
    - Effective use requires appropriate matching of the device to infant size, device location, and training.
    - Catheter securement using skin sutures was once considered the optimal choice but is now largely abandoned in NICUs and is no longer endorsed for most circumstances [24].
    - If a cyanoacrylate adhesive secured catheters must be removed early, only remove sufficient adhesive to ease catheter removal, residual adhesive can be safely left in place for natural separation [68].

- Once secured, protect the exit site and catheter with a dressing.
  - Sterile transparent materials with high moisture vapour transferability designed to fit infant anatomical contours are the preferred choice [24].
  - Cyanoacrylate adhesive can be applied to the dressing edges to improve dressing adhesion [69].
  - General guidance indicates that dressing changes are usually only required if the dressing becomes soiled, loosened, or excessive moisture collects. In such cases, reapply cyanoacrylate with every dressing change [24].
  - Surgical-ANTT® should be used for all dressing changes [24, 34, 39].

6.6   Complications

CVADs are associated with lower rates of complications than PVADs [10, 24, 44, 47]. However, this does not imply that CVADs are risk free. Numerous complications are reported in the literature (e.g., [7, 10, 16, 24, 44, 45, 52, 70–81]). Table 6.2 provides a summary and for clarity categorises these by timing (early, within the first 24 h, late onset, after 24 h) and where appropriate by device.

Exact figures for the incidences of different complications vary between research reports. This situation might reflect an absence of universally agreed categorisation or could be due to real differences in practice, but exact reasons for these differences are largely unknown. Whilst the list of potential complications is long, most are uncommon and only feature in occasional case reports. The most reported complications are catheter malposition and tip migration. The increased adoption of technological aids such as real-time ultrasound and IC-ECG combined with newer approaches for catheter securement will likely see reductions in this problem.

Complications arise from the interplay of modifiable procedural, unmodifiable, and potentially modifiable patient and organisational factors. For example, catheter tip migration can lead to the potentially fatal complication of cardiac tamponade. The condition reportedly occurs in 0.5–2% of infants with a CVAD and has a mortality of around 80% once established [74, 75, 78]. In the early 2000s, there was a cluster of reports concerning fatal cardiac tamponade [78]. Post investigation actions included:

- Greater diligence in periodically reviewing and confirming catheter tip location
- Reappraisal of the optimal catheter tip location
- Strategies for improved parent-healthcare communications
- Proposed changes in untoward event reporting and investigation processes
- Changes in how healthcare provider education and skill development are supervised.

Table 6.2 Early and late onset complications associated with neonatal CVAD

Early onset	Accidental vein perforation
	Accidental arterial puncture (or cannulation)
	Inability to thread or remove guidewire
	Catheter damage, fracture, or breakage
	Catheter dislodgement
	Catheter occlusion
	Infant pain, discomfort
	Infant physiologic instability—inability to tolerate procedure
	Difficulties transitioning from peripheral to central circulation (n-PICC\ECC)
	Air embolism
	Bleeding at insertion site
	Malposition of catheter tip
	Too shallow (not central circulation)
	Too deep (beyond target area)
	Deviation into non-target vessels
Later onset	Catheter malposition and tip migration post-procedure resulting in infiltration and extravasation with consequences like:
	Cardiac tamponade
	Cardiac arrhythmia
	Central vein perforation vascular erosion
	Pleural effusion
	Cardiac effusion
	Effusion into vertebral/spinal fluid spaces
	Vascular erosion
	Nerve injury
	Difficult removal post therapy—due to fibrin or bacterial plaque formation
	Localised skin surface infection
	Bloodstream infection
	Catheter dislodgement
	Catheter damage, fracture, or breakage
	Catheter occlusion
	Thrombosis
	Phlebitis (mechanical and chemical)

Table 6.3 Sources of central vascular infection

Extraluminal: Microbial ingress through catheter exit site (e.g., from the skin)
Intraluminal: Microbial ingress though infusion lines (e.g., hub contamination)
Secondary to other infection: For example, sepsis, pneumonia
Contaminated fluids: For example, during manufacture, storage, or local preparation

Newborn infants, particularly those born preterm constitute a high-risk patient group for infection. Infections, regardless of origin (Table 6.3) amongst infants are a problem because they affect survival and morbidity (pain, growth, stress, developmental outcomes). In addition, infections increase the length of hospitalisation and the use of health resources, together with increased complaint and litigation, and provider reputational harm.

Ideas about how to define, diagnose, and survey infection rates vary. Text Box 6.6 details some of the current ideas to illustrate this point.

Text Box 6.6 Practice Point: Infections—Definitions and Surveillance
- Healthcare-associated infection (HCAI)
  - A broad term referring to all types of infection that occur because of contact with healthcare services regardless of their setting [31]
- Hospital-acquired infection (HAI) (also known as nosocomial infection)
  - An important subset of HCAI, defined as infection developing in 48 hours or more after hospital admission [31, 82]
  - Clinically important subgroups of HAI include urinary, respiratory, and bloodstream infection
- Bloodstream infection (BSI)
  - Figures for BSI capture all causes of bloodstream infection
  - It is not generally used for surveillance but can be help differentiate areas of practice to focus upon to improve patient outcomes [24]
- Catheter-related bloodstream infection (CRBSI)
  - Generally defined by clinical symptoms of infection and diagnostic criteria that can confirm the catheter as the source of infection—positive blood and catheter tip culture is considered essential to support diagnosis [24]
- Central line associated bloodstream infection (CLABSI)
  - Commonly presented as the number of confirmed infections per 1000 catheter days [83]
  - Broadly defined as a primary BSI in a patient who has or had a central line within the 48 hour period before the development of the infection that is not attributable to any other cause [24, 83]
- Catheter-associated bloodstream infection (CABSI)
  - A term proposed by The Infusion Nurses Society (INS) [24] captures all vascular access related infection and navigates around the confused CLABSI data arising from international variations in definition, outcome reporting, use of the term, and data management
  - BSIs originating from PVAD or CVADs
- Hospital onset bacteraemia and fungaemia (HOB) [32, 73, 84]
  - Currently, HOB refers to a BSI diagnosed on or after the fourth day of hospitalisation confirmed by positive blood culture from a non-commensal organism
  - Further work is required to refine the definition and data management

Healthcare provider behaviour is an important contributory factor both limiting and exacerbating HAIs. Effective hand hygiene is the single most effective strategy [33]. Robust evidence indicates that a lack of compliance with best practices in hand hygiene or aseptic technique and failing to challenge others over poor practices are primary factors in the cause of acquired infection [31, 34, 35, 82]. The same sources highlight organisational issues such as poor standards of environmental cleaning, inadequate staffing for the workload, overcrowding, and badly designed patient flow process controls [31, 34, 35, 82].

6.6.1   CLABSI

Measures of CLABSI incidence vary internationally and between patient groups and healthcare settings. This variability is in part thought to be due to inconsistencies in definition, diagnosis, confirmation, outcome reporting, and data management [24]. Though some of the variation will reflect underlying environmental and patient risk, as well as practice variations [24]. Consequently, interpreting comparative CLABSI data over time and between different healthcare settings requires a degree of caution. CLABSI rates in NICUs have been reported as high as low double figures and sustained periods of zero [7, 10, 24, 37, 45, 66, 85, 86].

On occasion reported figures are affected by factors beyond the immediate influence of nurses or other healthcare providers. To illustrate, one study [52] reported a CLABSI rate of 0.58% (0.25/1000 catheter days), noting this was particularly low for the study site. In this study site, blood culture testing for confirmation of CLABSI required parents to pay. The authors comment that it might be that the low CLABSI rates reported in this study reflected parents' economic circumstances rather than a true reflection of infection rates. This explanation reveals one of the complexities encountered when making international comparisons.

Central vascular access infection is an important metric used for healthcare quality surveillance. Surveillance forms a foundation for understanding infection prevalence and how effective individual infection prevention strategies are. In some jurisdictions, these measures are used to inform funding decisions. This can result in perverse incentive for changing practice which might not necessarily be in patients' best interests. For example, the growing trend for switching from central to peripheral devices, despite clear evidence for higher rates of complication with these devices [85].

Despite its limitations, CLABSI rates can be a useful measure when reporting on the effectiveness of locally devised interventions designed to reduce infection. Measures aimed at preventing CLABSI can be divided into technical and socio-behavioural measures.

- Technical measures
  - Include: determining optimal chemical compositions for skin disinfection and incorporating materials and designs to prevent infection, for example.

- Socio-behavioural measures
  - Include: focused education, teamworking, evidence-based bundles and check-lists, feedback and debriefing, empowering staff and parents to challenge others, for example.

Using the MST for n-PICC/ECC insertion is associated with reductions in CLABSI incidence [45, 86]. Reasons for this association are unclear. Speculatively, it might relate to the combined effects of greater first-attempt successful insertion, resulting in fewer episodes of skin breakage, reduced vein trauma and blood loss [46]. Arguably, it might also reflect greater team cohesion and teamworking following multi-professional education and training, factors known to directly influence CLABSI rates [87, 88].

van Rens et al. [89] found that adding a preassembled closed intravenous set to an n-PICC/ECC care bundle was associated with reduced CLABSI. However, this finding does not suggest that closed systems are a panacea for CLABSI prevention regardless of contextual and situational factors. In this study unit, the incidence was already below international comparators and compliance with existing CLABSI prevention care bundles was near 100% (internal audit data). Rather the inference from this result is that closed systems can lead to incrementally better outcomes but only if all preexisting CLABSI prevention measures are in place and there is good compliance with their implementation.

Focused quality improvement (QI) initiatives using evidence-based care bundles can bring about statistically significant reductions in CLABSI (e.g., [37, 38]). In one NICU, Bierlere and colleagues [38] introduced a new CVAD dressing and maintenance bundle. This bundle introduced the use of cyanoacrylate tissue adhesive for exit site sealing and catheter securement combined with more robust approaches to hand hygiene and aseptic technique compliance. The CLABSI incidence declined from 8.4 to 1.8 per 1000 catheter days over the study period [38]. There is a substantial body of quasi-experimental research evidence supporting the effectiveness of care bundles in reducing CLABSI incidences amongst NICU patients. However, a clear understanding of which elements are essential or most effective is lacking and further research is required to clarify this matter [37].

Research reports about the efficacy of using miconazole and rifampicin antimicrobial coated n-PICC/ECCs to prevent CLABSI are generally inconclusive [90–92]. Wu et al. [91] analysed two randomised controlled trials and seven retro or prospective studies involving a total of 51,373 patients. Their analysis found no statistically significant association between using n-PICC/ECCs coated with antimicrobials and CLABSI risk in whole group or subgroup analyses. Speculatively, the lack of supportive data concerning the effectiveness of antimicrobial coatings might be ascribed to several factors. For example, misplaced assumptions about the causation of CLABSI, methodological weaknesses, differing diagnostic and surveillance criteria or interactions between confounding variables, such as:

- Different care settings
  - Critical care, primary care or home, for instance

- Different background risk factors for BSI
  - Dominant environmental bacterial strains, choice of insertion technique, compliance with infection prevention bundles, etc.
- Different patient populations
  - Adult, adolescent, young children, neonatal
- Patients with different medical conditions
  - Incorrect choice of coatings, chronic illnesses, cancer treatments, immuno-suppression, for example.

Likely more nuanced research using appropriately powered study methodologies will provide more definitive answers to guide practice (Text Box 6.7).

Text Box 6.7 Practice Point: Reducing Infection Risk, Things That Help
- Ensuring adequate staffing and skill mix for the workload.
- Using a team approach for all aspects of vascular access.
- Consideration of unmodifiable patient characteristics (e.g., immune status, skin condition, protein calorie malnutrition) incorporated into vascular access planning.
- Planning to avoid unduly prolonged NICU stays.
- Audited 100% compliance with good hand hygiene practices and organisational standards for infection prevention and control precautions.
- Audited good compliance with evidence-based care bundles for insertion, using and removing CVADs.
- Skin preparation with chlorhexidine gluconate and alcohol solutions or applicators.
- Maximal sterile precautions during insertion and accessing lines and catheters.
- Avoidance of insertion sites with a high risk of contamination.
- Using minimal number of lumens required for effective therapy.
- Effective exit site sealing, catheter securement, and dressing.
- Having systems in place to routinely collect comprehensive vascular access data to enable clinical audit and root cause analysis if adverse events occur.
- Removing devices when no longer essential—no CVAD no CLABSI!
- And most importantly: *communicate* with the team, including parents.

6.7   Promoting Comfort, Relieving Pain, and Involving Parents

Low gestational age remains the clearest indicator for poor neurodevelopmental outcomes. Evidence indicates that infants, especially those born preterm are vulnerable to adverse developmental effects from early life pain and stress [93, 94].

Consequently, taking action to reduce pain experience (number of occasions and severity) whilst indicative of compassionate humane care can also improve developmental outcomes.

Efficacious strategies for reducing infant stress and promoting comfort like skin-to-skin contact (kangaroo care) are largely contraindicated during most CVAD insertions. This is due to the need for sterility, precise positioning, and avoidance of infant movement. However, other facets of neurodevelopmentally supportive care interventions can be readily used. Examples (see Chap. 4, Fig. 4.1) include swaddling, containment holding, parent body odour, pre-procedural oral sucrose solutions or breastmilk, non-nutritive sucking, and parent voice [95–100]. Interventions such as these can be readily applied during CVAD insertion without unduly affecting insertion processes.

Two examples: Mothers' breastmilk odour is known to be comforting [99, 100]; it is a simple matter to ensure that a small amount of breastmilk is placed in proximity to the infant's head. Secondly, providing infants with low volume audio recordings of their parent's speech or singing could provide opportunity for parents to be vicariously present. Doing these would expose the infant's olfactory system to a comforting odour and their auditory system to familiar human voices. Furthermore, it could help to ensure that parents feel involved and reassure them that their infant's comfort is being prioritised. The incorporation of non-pharmacological interventions into a CVAD insertion care bundle can ensure consistent use and care equity.

To ensure patient safety during CICC and FICC (tunnelled and non-tunnelled), insertion pharmacological analgesia and/or conscious sedation or surgical anaesthesia are required. Though many drug options are unlicensed for use in neonates' treatment, monographs suggesting options and dosing regimens are available. In this context, common medications for sedation, acute analgesia, and short-term procedural anaesthesia include midazolam, synthetic opioids (fentanyl 'family'), ketamine, and propofol. For detailed and specific advice on safe use, dosing regimens, precautions, and hazards, nurses and prescribers should consult local hospital formularies, pharmacists, and other authoritative sources (e.g., British National Formulary for Children, (BNFC), https://bnfc.nice.org.uk).

6.7.1   Parent Involvement

NICU stress experiences significantly affect parent mental health and satisfaction with care [101]. More psychological stress leads to greater mental health adversity and reduced levels of satisfaction with care [101]. Feelings of stress, being an outsider and powerlessness over control of events are common amongst NICU parents. Nurses are well placed to positively affect parent-NICU staff relationships and help them navigate their time in the NICU [102–105].

In contrast to PVAD insertion when parents can play an active role, the restrictions around CVAD (maintaining sterility, managing sedation or anaesthesia) preclude their presence from much of the procedure. This situation can heighten parental anxiety and requires timely sensitive explanation to mitigate its effects.

Overly medico-technological explanations or inconsistencies in language can be inhibitive to parental understanding. This can create a sense of isolation, confusion, and can lead to parental complaint [104, 106, 107].

In practice, using different descriptive terms or local colloquialisms for the same device can lead to misunderstanding. In addition, referring to the insertion itself as 'a simple procedure just like having an IV catheter' might not prepare parents for the reality of seeing an n-PICC/ECC in scalp vein or tunnelled FICC in their infant. Nurses should ensure that any verbal explanations use consistent readily understandable language and terms. Evidence indicates verbal explanations supported by written and visual materials, and peer support is considered the most helpful [108]. In reality, the nature of parental communications around vascular access will be influenced by the context of insertion. For example, during an emergency or when managing an unstable infant, discussions around clinical management concerns might have greater priority.

Opportunities to increase partnership working during CVAD insertion might on first inspection seem limited compared to PVAD insertion. Nonetheless, there are things nurses can do to increase these opportunities. Two examples include: firstly encouraging and providing emotional and practical support for parents to engage in shared dialogue during scheduled multidisciplinary ward rounds can provide opportunities for parents to feel their voice is heard. Secondly, and admittedly not universally promoted it is considered feasible in some NICUs to make provision for a suitably prepared and briefed parent wearing the correct personal protective equipment to be present during the n-PICC insertion procedure. Doing this can address deeply seated parental anxieties and foster increased trust in nurse–parent relationships. Furthermore, parental presence, voice, and touch (away from the sterile field) can add to existing comfort promoting measures.

6.8   Concluding Remarks

Infusion therapy using central vasculature routes is important and often the most reliable therapeutic options in NICUs. Their insertion and use are emerging as an important area of practice for nurses in vascular access teams or advanced practice roles. This chapter has considered the range of venous CVADs commonly encountered in neonatal care. Successful insertion of CVADs requires a team approach and a command of high level skills. The modified MST is described alongside consideration of a range of common and rare complications. Chief amongst these are the prevention and surveillance strategies used around bloodstream infection.

At first inspection, CVAD insertion and use might preclude parental involvement. However, there are opportunities to increase parental integration into care beyond current levels. Some of those highlighted in this chapter include applying existing neuroprotective and developmentally supportive interventions more commonly seen in peripheral vascular access.

Key Points

- The selection of which CVAD-n-PICC/ECC, CICC, or FICC (tunnelled and non-tunnelled) to use should be determined by a thorough and systematic pre-procedural assessment of vein suitability, consideration of patient characteristics, and therapeutic need.
- Consideration of non-pharmacological and pharmacological pain management interventions needs to be factored into care. In addition, for some CVADs, the selection of safe approaches for sedation and anaesthesia needs to be incorporating into care.
- Surgical-ANTT® is mandatory during central catheter insertion.
- Evidence about the optimal securement and dressing of neonatal CVADs is incomplete. But the safety and efficacy of cyanoacrylate tissue adhesives, engineered devices, and integrated dressings used alone or in combination are convincing.
- Nurses need to be vigilant about the range of common and rare early and late onset complications associated with CVAD insertion and understand the contribution of preventative strategies.
- Bloodstream infection is a major concern during CVAD use and measures to prevent infection are essential. These measures include universal compliance with handwashing, effective skin disinfection, Surgical-ANTT®, and evidence-based care bundles.
- Due to the need to maintain asepsis, complexities and technical nature of CVAD insertion parents can feel excluded. However, establishing measures to ensure adequate explanations and reassurance promotes greater parental involvement such as opportunities to provide skin-to-skin contact, which can help alleviate these feelings.

Reflective Activity Managing Complications During PICC Insertion

Read the following case related to an episode of vascular access and consider your responses to the reflective questions at the end.

You are an NICU nurse caring for Stephan, a clinically stable preterm infant born at 27 weeks gestation. He had an n-PICC/ECC inserted in his left arm for administering parenteral nutrition a few hours previously. Insertion was reported as difficult with resistance felt (but overcome) when making the transition from the peripheral to central circulation. Catheter tip location was confirmed post-procedure, and the catheter secured and dressed using your unit's usual procedures. On examination of the catheter exit site though the transparent dressing, you observe signs of swelling and discoloration at the site.

Considering the above case and your reading in this chapter, reflect on your answers to the following questions:

1. What immediate actions would you take to address this finding?
   (a) Consider how would you prioritise these actions. Think, would you remove the n-PICC/ECC at this moment?
   (b) Consider how you would you ensure the well-being and comfort of Stephan and manage his vulnerabilities, pain, or distress.
2. How would you and what would you communicate about your observations and actions regarding this situation to others?
   (a) Think about how you might use an appropriate structured communication tool (SBAR, ISBAR, I-PASS, etc.) and who you would need to communicate with—your immediate supervisor and the wider healthcare team and Stephan's parents.
3. How would you and your unit set about investigating and addressing factors or causes that might have contributed to this problem?
   (a) Think about the formal notification, escalation, and investigative processes for untoward events in your NICU and your role in root cause analyses (RCA).

References

1. Barone G, Pittiruti M. Epicutaneo-caval catheters in neonates: new insights and new suggestions from the recent literature. J Vasc Access. 2019;21(6):805–9. https://doi.org/10.1177/1129729819891546.
2. Pittiruti M, Van Boxtel T, Scoppettuolo G, Carr P, Konstantinou E, Ortiz Miluy G, et al. European recommendations on the proper indication and use of peripheral venous access devices (the ERPIUP consensus): a WoCoVA project. J Vasc Access. 2023;24(1):165–82. https://doi.org/10.1177/11297298211023274.
3. Barone G, D'Andrea V, Ancora G, Cresi F, Maggio L, Capasso A, et al. The neonatal DAV-expert algorithm: a GAVeCeLT/GAVePed consensus for the choice of the most appropriate venous access in newborns. Eur J Pediatr. 2023;182(8):3385–95. https://doi.org/10.1007/s00431-023-04984-4.
4. Ullman AJ, Bernstein SJ, Brown E, Aiyagari R, Doellman D, Faustino EVS, et al. The Michigan appropriateness guide for intravenous catheters in pediatrics: min-iMAGIC. Pediatrics. 2020;145(Suppl 3):S269–84. https://doi.org/10.1542/peds.2019-3474I.
5. van Rens MFPT, Bayoumi MA, van de Hoogen A, Francia ALV, Cabanillas IJ, van Loon FHJ, et al. The ABBA project (assess better before access): a retrospective, cross-sectional study of neonatal intravascular device outcomes. Front Pediatr. 2022;10:10.980725. https://doi.org/10.3389/fped.2022.980725.
6. Paterson RS, Chopra V, Brown E, Kleidon TM, Cooke M, Rickard CM, et al. Selection and insertion of vascular access devices in pediatrics: a systematic review. Pediatrics. 2020;45(Suppl. 3):S243–68. https://doi.org/10.1542/peds.2019-3474H.
7. British Association of Perinatal Medicine, (BAPM). Use of central venous catheters in neonates a framework for practice. London: BAPM; 2018.

8. D'Andrea V, Prontera G, Rubortone SA, Pezza L, Pinna G, Barone G, et al. Umbilical venous catheter update: a narrative review including ultrasound and training. Front Pediatr. 2022;9:774705. https://doi.org/10.3389/fped.2021.774705.

9. Madar J, Roehr CR, Ainsworth S, Ersdal H, Morley C, Rüdiger M, et al. European Resuscitation Council guidelines 2021: newborn resuscitation and support of transition of infants at birth. Resuscitation. 2021;161:291–326. https://doi.org/10.1016/j.resuscitation.2021.02.014.

10. Sharpe EI, Curry S, Mason-Wyckoff M. Peripherally inserted central catheters: guideline for practice, vol. 24. 4th ed. Chicago: National Association of Neonatal Nurses; 2022. https://nann.mycrowdwisdom.com/cw/course-details?entryId=10902832. Accessed 12 August 2024. p. 313.

11. Uygun I. Peripherally inserted central catheter in neonates: a safe and easy technique. J Pediatr Surg. 2016;51(1):188–91. https://doi.org/10.1016/j.jpedsurg.2015.08.008.

12. Barone G, Pittiruti M, Ancora G, Vento G, Tota F, D'Andrea V. Centrally inserted central catheters in preterm neonates with weight below 1500 g by ultrasound-guided access to the brachio-cephalic vein. J Vasc Access. 2021;22(3):344–52. https://doi.org/10.1177/1129729820940174.

13. Pittiruti M, Celentano D, Barone G, D'Andrea V, Annetta MG, Conti G. A GAVeCeLT bundle for central venous catheterization in neonates and children: a prospective clinical study on 729 cases. J Vasc Access. 2023;24(6):1477–88. https://doi.org/10.1177/11297298221074472.

14. Brescia F, Pittiruti M, Spencer TR, Dawson RB. The SIP protocol update: eight strategies, incorporating Rapid Peripheral Vein Assessment (RaPeVA), to minimize complications associated with peripherally inserted central catheter insertion. J Vasc Access. 2022;25:5. https://doi.org/10.1177/11297298221099838.

15. August D, Ullman AJ, Rickard CM, New K. Peripheral intravenous catheter practices in Australian and New Zealand neonatal units: a cross-sectional survey. J Neonat Nurs. 2019;25(5):240–4. https://doi.org/10.1016/j.jnn.2019.03.002.

16. Brescia F, Pittiruti M, Ostroff M, Spencer TR, Dawson RB. The SIC protocol: a seven-step strategy to minimize complications potentially related to the insertion of centrally inserted central catheters. J Vasc Access. 2023;24(2):185–90. https://doi.org/10.1177/11297298211036002.

17. Spencer TR, Pittiruti M. Rapid Central Vein Assessment (RaCeVA): a systematic, standardized approach for ultrasound assessment before central venous catheterization. J Vasc Access. 2019;20(3):239–49. https://doi.org/10.1177/1129729818804718.

18. Brescia F, Pittiruti M, Ostroff M, Biasucci DG. Rapid femoral vein assessment (RaFeVA): a systematic protocol for ultrasound evaluation of the veins of the lower limb, so to optimize the insertion of femorally inserted central catheters. J Vasc Access. 2021;22(6):863–72. https://doi.org/10.1177/1129729820965063.

19. Breschan C, Platzer M, Jost R, Stettner H, Feigl G, Likar R. Ultrasound-guided supraclavicular cannulation of the brachiocephalic vein in infants: a retrospective analysis of a case series. Pediatr Anesth. 2012;22(11):1062–7. https://doi.org/10.1111/j.1460-9592.2012.03923.x.

20. Breschan C, Graf G, Jost R, Stettner H, Feigl G, Neuwersch S, et al. A retrospective analysis of the clinical effectiveness of supraclavicular, ultrasound-guided brachiocephalic vein cannulations in preterm infants. Anesth. 2018;128:38–43. https://doi.org/10.1097/ALN.0000000000001871.

21. Breschan C, Graf G, Arneitz C, Stettner H, Feigl G, Neuwersch S, et al. Feasibility of the ultrasound-guided supraclavicular cannulation of the brachiocephalic vein in very small weight infants: a case series. Pediatr Anesth. 2020;30(8):928–33. https://doi.org/10.1111/pan.13928.

22. Ostroff MD, Moureau N, Pittiruti M. Rapid assessment of vascular exit site and tunneling options (RAVESTO): a new decision tool in the management of the complex vascular access patients. J Vasc Access. 2023;24(2):311–7. https://doi.org/10.1177/11297298211034306.

23. Barone G, D'Andrea V, Vento G, Pittiruti M. A systematic ultrasound evaluation of the diameter of deep veins in the newborn: results and implications for clinical practice. Neonatology. 2019;115(4):335–40. https://doi.org/10.1159/000496848.

24. Nickel B, Gorski L, Kleidon T, Kyes A, DeVries M, Keogh S, et al. Infusion therapy standards of practice. 9th ed. J Inf Nurs. 2024;47(1S):S1–285. https://doi.org/10.1097/NAN.0000000000000532.

25. Sharp R, Cummings M, Fielder A, Mikocka-Walus A, Grech C, Esterman A. The catheter to vein ratio and rates of symptomatic venous thromboembolism in patients with a peripherally inserted central catheter (PICC): a prospective cohort study. Int J Nurs Stud. 2015;52(3):677–85. https://doi.org/10.1016/j.ijnurstu.2014.12.002.

26. Sharp R, Carr P, Childs J, Scullion A, Young M, Flynn T, et al. Catheter to vein ratio and risk of peripherally inserted central catheter (PICC)-associated thrombosis according to diagnostic group: a retrospective cohort study. BMJ Open. 2021;11:e045895. https://doi.org/10.1136/bmjopen-2020-045895.

27. Nifong TP, McDevitt TJ. The effect of catheter to vein ratio on blood flow rates in a simulated model of peripherally inserted central venous catheters. Chest. 2011;140(1):P48–53. https://doi.org/10.1378/chest.10-2637.

28. Osborn NK, Baron TH. The history of the 'French' gauge. Gastrointest Endosc. 2006;63(3):461–2. https://doi.org/10.1016/j.gie.2005.11.019.

29. Poll JS. The story of the gauge. Anaesth. 1999;5496:575–81. https://doi.org/10.1046/j.1365-2044.1999.00895.x.

30. Spagnuolo F, Maietta A, Pugliese U, Lettieri E, Minopoli F, Coppola N, et al. Systematic application of SICA-PED protocol for central venous catheterization in neonates: a prospective clinical study on 104 cases. J Vasc Access. 2024; https://doi.org/10.1177/11297298241239998.

31. National Institute for Health and Care Excellence (NICE). Healthcare-associated infections: prevention and control (PH36). London: NICE; 2011, 2024. www.nice.org.uk/guidance/ph36. Accessed 12 August 2024.

32. Schrank GM, Snyder GM, Leekha S. Hospital-onset bacteremia and fungemia: examining healthcare-associated infections prevention through a wider lens. Antimicrob Steward Healthc Epidemiol. 2023;3(1):e198. https://doi.org/10.1017/ash.2023.486.

33. World Health Organisation (WHO). Save lives, clean your hands. A guide to the implementation of the WHO multimodal hand hygiene improvement strategy. https://iris.who.int/bitstream/handle/10665/44196/9789241598606_eng.pdf?sequence=1. Accessed 12 August 2024.

34. Centers for Disease Control and Prevention, (CDC). CDC's core infection prevention and control practices for safe healthcare delivery in all settings, 29 November 2022. https://www.cdc.gov/infectioncontrol/guidelines/core-practices/index.html. Accessed 12 August 2024.

35. National Health Service (NHS) England. National infection prevention and control manual for England, V2.4. London: NHS England; 2023.

36. Rowley S, Clare S. Guidance document. Standardizing the critical clinical competency of aseptic, sterile, and clean techniques with a single international standard: aseptic non touch technique (ANTT®). Mount Royal: Association for Vascular Access; 2019.

37. Payne V, Hall M, Prieto J, Johnson M. Care bundles to reduce central line-associated bloodstream infections in the neonatal unit: a systematic review and meta-analysis. Arch Dis Child Fetal Neonat Ed. 2018;103(5):F422–9. https://doi.org/10.1136/archdischild-2017-313362.

38. Bierlaire S, Danhaive O, Carkeek K, Piersigilli F. How to minimize central line-associated bloodstream infections in a neonatal intensive care unit: a quality improvement intervention based on a retrospective analysis and the adoption of an evidence-based bundle. Eur J Pediatr. 2021;180(2):449–60. https://doi.org/10.1007/s00431-020-03844-9.

39. ANTT® procedure guidelines. https://www.antt.org/antt-procedure-guidelines.html. Accessed 12 August 2024.

40. Khurana S, Saini SS, Sundaram V, Dutta S, Kumar P. Reducing healthcare-associated infections in neonates by standardizing and improving compliance to aseptic non-touch techniques: a quality improvement approach. Indian Pediatr. 2018;55(9):748–52. https://doi.org/10.1007/s13312-018-1373-6.
41. Barone G, Pittiruti M, Biasucci DG, Elisei D, Lacobone E, La Greca A, et al. Neo-ECHOTIP: a structured protocol for ultrasound-based tip navigation and tip location during placement of central venous access devices in neonates. J Vasc Access. 2022;23(5):679–88. https://doi.org/10.1177/11297298211007703.
42. Spagnuolo F. Global use of ultrasound in newborn vascular access: RA. CE. VA: implantation and management of complications. J Ultrasound. 2023;27:397. https://doi.org/10.1007/s40477-023-00813-4.
43. Athikarisamy SE, Veldman A, Malhotra A, Wong F. Using a modified Seldinger technique is an effective way of placing femoral venous catheters in critically ill infants. Acta Paediatr. 2015;104(6):e241–6. https://doi.org/10.1111/apa.12973.
44. Hugill K, Van Rens M. Inserting central lines via the peripheral circulation in neonates. Brit J Nurs. 2020;29(19):S12–8. https://doi.org/10.12968/bjon.2020.29.19.S12.
45. van Rens MFPT, Hugill K, van den Lee R, Francia ALV, van Loon FHJ, Bayoumi MAA. Comparing conventional and modified Seldinger technique using a micro insertion kit for PICC placement in neonates: a retrospective cohort study. 2024;12:1395395. https://doi.org/10.3389/fped.2024.1395395.
46. Callejas A, Osiovich H, Ting JY. Use of peripherally inserted central catheters (PICC) via scalp veins in neonates. J Matern Fetal Neonat Med. 2016;29(21):34–8. https://doi.org/10.3109/14767058.2016.1139567.
47. Song IK, Kim EH, Lee JH, Jang YE, Kim HS, Kim JT. Seldinger vs modified Seldinger techniques for ultrasound-guided central venous catheterization in neonates: a randomised controlled trial. Brit J Anaesth. 2018;121(6):1332–7.
48. Wald M, Happel CM, Kirchner L, Jeitler V, Sasse M, Wessel A. Modified Seldinger technique for 2-French peripherally inserted central venous catheters. Arc Dis Child. 2008;93(supp 2): Ps368.
49. MacLeod R, Gibb J, MacLeod R, Elanjikal Z. 55 modified Seldinger technique for neonatal peripherally inserted central catheter placement. BMJ Paediatr Open. 2021;5:35. https://doi.org/10.1136/bmjpo-2021-RCPCH.35.
50. Pereira HP, Secco IL, Arrue AM, Pontes L, Danski MTR. Implementation of modified Seldinger technology for percutaneous catheterization in critically ill newborns. Rev Esc Enferm USP. 2023;57:e20220347. https://doi.org/10.1590/1980-220X-REEUSP-2022-0347en.
51. Gibb JJC, MacLeod R, Mahoney L, Elanjikal Z. Modified Seldinger technique for neonatal epicutaneo-caval catheter insertion: a non-randomised retrospective study. J Vasc Access. 2023;24(4):780–5. https://doi.org/10.1177/11297298211054637.
52. Wu Y, Yan J, Tang M, Hu Y, Wan X, Li X, et al. A review of neonatal peripherally inserted central venous catheters in extremely or very low birthweight infants based on a 3-year clinical practice: complication incidences and risk factors. Front Pediatr. 2022;10:10. https://doi.org/10.3389/fped.2022.987512.
53. Pettit J. Technological advances for PICC placement and management. Adv Neonat Care. 2007;7(34):122–31. https://doi.org/10.1097/01.ANC.0000278210.18639.fd.
54. Suell JV, Meshkati M, Juliano C, Groves A. Real-time point-of-care ultrasound-guided correction of PICC line placement by external manipulation of the upper extremity. Arch Dis Child Fetal Neonat Ed. 2020;105(1):F25. https://doi.org/10.1136/archdischild-2019-317610.
55. Spencer TR. Repositioning of central venous access devices using a high-flow flush technique—a clinical practice and cost review. J Vasc Access. 2017;18(5):419–25.
56. Wang D, Niu F, Gao H, Yu M, Li Y, Xu L, et al. Influence of guide wire removal on tip location in peripherally inserted central catheters (PICCs): a retrospective cross-sectional study. BMJ Open. 2019;9(10):e027278. https://doi.org/10.1136/bmjopen-2018-027278.

57. van Rens MFPT, Paramban R, Francia ALV, Chandra P, Mahmah MA, Thome UH, et al. Evaluation of a diluted lipid emulsion solution as a lubricant for improved peripherally inserted central catheter guidewire removal in a neonatal population. BMC Pediatr. 2022;22(1):71. https://doi.org/10.1186/s12887-022-03119-2.

58. Chen I-L, Ou-Yang M-C, Chen F-S, Chung M-Y, Chen CC, Liu Y-C, et al. The equations of the inserted length of percutaneous central venous catheters on neonates in NICU. Pediatr Neonat. 2019;60(3):305–10. https://doi.org/10.1016/j.pedneo.2018.07.011.

59. Singh Y, Tissot C, Fraga MV, Yousef N, Cortes RG, Lopez J, et al. International evidence-based guidelines on point of care ultrasound (POCUS) for critically ill neonates and children issued by the POCUS Working Group of the European Society of Paediatric and Neonatal Intensive Care (ESPNIC). Crit Care. 2020;24(1):65. https://doi.org/10.1186/s13054-020-2787-9.

60. Barone G, Pittiruti M, D'Andrea V. Ultrasound-guided catheter tip location in neonatal central venous access. Focus on well-defined protocols and proper ultrasound training. J Pediatr. 2022;247:181. https://doi.org/10.1016/j.jpeds.2022.05.035.

61. Capasso A, Mastroianni R, Passariello A, Palma M, Messina F, Ansalone A, et al. The intra-cavitary electrocardiography method for positioning the tip of epicutaneous cava catheter in neonates: pilot study. J Vasc Access. 2018;19(6):542–7. https://doi.org/10.1177/1129729818761292.

62. Xiao AQ, Sun J, Zhu LH, Liao ZY, Shen P, Zhao LL, et al. Effectiveness of intracavitary electrocardiogram-guided peripherally inserted central catheter tip placement in premature infants: a multicentre pre-post intervention study. Eur J Pediatr. 2020;179(3):439–46. https://doi.org/10.1007/s00431-019-03524-3.

63. HB Fuller. SecurePortIV: indication for use (IFU). SPI-IFU01-1903. (June 2019). www.SPIVTraining.com. Accessed 12 January 2025.

64. D'Andrea V, Barone G, Pezza L, Prontera G, Vento G, Pittiruti M. Securement of central venous catheters by subcutaneously anchored sutureless devices in neonates. J Matern Fetal Neonat Med. 2021;35(25):6747–50. https://doi.org/10.1080/14767058.2021.1922377.

65. Spencer TR. Securing vascular access devices. Am Nurse Today. 2018;13(9):29–31.

66. van Rens MFPT, Nimeri AMA, Spencer TR, Hugill K, Francia ALV, Olukade TO, et al. Cyanoacrylate securement in neonatal PICC use, a 4-year observational study. Adv Neonat Care. 2021;22(3):270–9. https://doi.org/10.1097/ANC.0000000000000963.

67. D'Andrea V, Pezza L, Barone G, Prontera G, Pittiruti M, Vento G. Use of cyanoacrylate glue for the sutureless securement of epicutaneo-caval catheters in neonates. J Vasc Access. 2022;23(5):801–4. https://doi.org/10.1177/11297298211008103.

68. Hugill K, van Rens MFPT, Alderman A, Kaczmarek L, Lund C, Paradis A. Safe and effective removal of cyanoacrylate vascular access catheter securement adhesive in neonates. Front Pediatr. 2023;11(1237648):1–5. https://doi.org/10.3389/fped.2023.1237648.

69. Zhang S, Price N, Guido A. Addition of cyanoacrylate adhesive improves the strength of catheter securement and integrity of transparent dressing: results from an in vitro test model. J Vasc Access. 2023;25:1238. https://doi.org/10.1177/11297298231159177.

70. Rocha G, Soares P, Pissarra S, Soares H, Costa S, Henriques-Coelho T, et al. Vascular access in neonates. Minerva Pediatr. 2017;69(1):72–82. https://doi.org/10.23736/S0026-4946.16.04348-6.

71. Diniz ERS, de Araújo Santos Camargo JD, de Medeiros KS, da Silva RAR, Cobucci RN, Roncalli AG. Risk factors for the development of peripherally inserted central catheter-related bloodstream infection in neonates: prospective cohort study. J Neonat Nurs. 2023;29(2):387–92. https://doi.org/10.1016/j.jnn.2022.08.006.

72. Perme T. Central lines and their complications in neonates: a case report and literature review. Children (Basel). 2023;11(1):26. https://doi.org/10.3390/children11010026.

73. Yu KC, Ye G, Edwards JR, Gupta V, Benin AL, Ai C, et al. Hospital-onset bacteremia and fungemia: an evaluation of predictors and feasibility of benchmarking comparing two risk-adjusted models among 267 hospitals. Infect Cont Hosp Epidemiol. 2022;43(10):1317–25. https://doi.org/10.1017/ice.2022.211.

74. Zareef R, Anka M, Hatab T, El Rassi I, Yunis K, Bitar F, et al. Tamponade and massive pleural effusions secondary to peripherally inserted central catheter in neonates-a complication to be aware of. Front Cardiovasc Med. 2023;10:1092814. https://doi.org/10.3389/fcvm.2023.1092814.

75. Zarkesh MR, Haghjoo M. Neonatal cardiac tamponade, a life-threatening complication secondary to peripherally inserted central catheter: a case report. J Med Case Rep. 2022;16(1):305. https://doi.org/10.1186/s13256-022-03506-4.

76. Blackwood BP, Farrow KN, Kim S, Hunter CJ. Peripherally inserted central catheters complicated by vascular erosion in neonates. J Parenter Enter Nutr. 2016;40(6):890–5. https://doi.org/10.1177/0148607115574000.

77. Ruikka JL, Acun C, Karnati S. Entrapped peripherally inserted central catheter due to fibrin sheath in a neonate with noninvasive extraction and review of literature. J Neonat Perinat Med. 2022;15(2):383–6. https://doi.org/10.3233/NPM-210830.

78. Department of Health (DOH). Review of the deaths of four babies due to cardiac tamponade associated with the presence of a central venous catheter. London: DOH; 2001. https://webarchive.nationalarchives.gov.uk/ukgwa/20130107105354/http:/www.dh.gov.uk/prod_consum_dh/groups/dh_digitalassets/@dh/@en/documents/digitalasset/dh_4058241.pdf. Accessed 12 August 2024

79. Pettit J. Assessment of infants with peripherally inserted central catheters: part 1. Detecting the most frequently occurring complications. Adv Neonat Care. 2002;2(6):304–15. https://doi.org/10.1053/adnc.2002.36826.

80. Pettit J. Assessment of infants with peripherally inserted central catheters: part 2. Detecting less frequently occurring complications. Adv Neonat Care. 2003;3(1):14–26. https://doi.org/10.1053/adnc.2003.50011.

81. Farag MM, Ghazal HAER, Radwan MM, El-Sayed NS. Catheters linked thrombosis in neonates: a single center observational study. Ital J Pediatr. 2024;50(1):147. https://doi.org/10.1186/s13052-024-01708-8.

82. Loveday HP, Wilson JA, Pratt RJ, Golsorkhi M, Tingle A, Bak A, et al. epic3: national evidence-based guidelines for preventing healthcare-associated infections in NHS hospitals in England. J Hosp Infect. 2014;86(Suppl 1):S1–S70. https://doi.org/10.1016/S0195-6701(13)60012-2.

83. Centers for Disease Control and Prevention, (CDC). The 2019 *National and State healthcare-associated infections (HAI) progress report*. 2019. https://www.cdc.gov/hai/data/portal/progress-report.html

84. Leekha S, Robinson GL, Jacob JT, Fridkin S, Shane A, Sick-Samuels A, et al. Evaluation of hospital-onset bacteraemia and fungaemia in the USA as a potential healthcare quality measure: a cross-sectional study. BMJ Qual Saf. 2024;33(8):487–98. https://doi.org/10.1136/bmjqs-2023-016831.

85. van Rens MFPT, van Boxtel AJH, Mermel LA. Comment on: Central-line-associated bloodstream infection (CLABSI) burden among Dutch neonatal intensive care units. J Hosp Infect. 2024;150:174–5. https://doi.org/10.1016/j.jhin.2024.03.024.

86. Arnts IJJ, Schrijvers NM, van der Flier M, Groenewoud JMM, Antonius T, Liem KD. Central line bloodstream infections can be reduced in newborn infants using the modified Seldinger technique and care bundles of preventative measures. Acta Paediatr. 2015;104(4):e152–7. https://doi.org/10.1111/apa.12915.

87. Bayoumi MAA, Van Rens MFP, Chandra P, Francia ALV, D'Souza S, George M, et al. Effect of implementing an epicutaneo-caval catheter team in neonatal intensive care unit. J Vasc Access. 2021;22(2):243–53. https://doi.org/10.1177/1129729820928182.

88. Krein SL, Kuhn L, Ratz D, Chopra V. Use of designated nurse PICC teams and CLABSI prevention practices among U.S. hospitals: a survey-based study. J Patient Saf. 2019;15(4):293–5. https://doi.org/10.1097/PTS.0000000000000246.

89. van Rens MFPT, Hugill K, Francia ALV, Mahmah MA, Al Shadad ABJ, Chiuco IC, et al. Closed intravenous system for central vascular access: a difference maker for CLABSI rates in neonates? J Vasc Access. 2022;24:1–8. https://doi.org/10.1177/11297298221085480.

90. Gilbert R, Brown M, Rainford N, Donohue C, Fraser C, Sinha A, et al. Antimicrobial-impregnated central venous catheters for prevention of neonatal bloodstream infection (PREVAIL): an open-label, parallel-group, pragmatic, randomised controlled trial. Lancet Child Adolesc Health. 2019;3(6):381–90. https://doi.org/10.1016/S2352-4642(19)301142.

91. Wu Y, Lei Y, Wang B, Feng B. Efficacy of antimicrobial peripherally inserted central catheters in line-associated bloodstream infections: a systematic review and meta-analysis. Am J Inf Control. 2023;51(12):1425–9. https://doi.org/10.1016/j.ajic.2023.04.163.

92. Bayoumi MAA, van Rens MFPT, Chandra P, Masry A, D'Souza S, Khalil AM, et al. Does the antimicrobial-impregnated peripherally inserted central catheter decrease the CLABSI rate in neonates? Results from a retrospective cohort study. Front Pediatr. 2022;10:1012800. https://doi.org/10.3389/fped.2022.1012800.

93. van Dokkum NH, de Kroon MLA, Reijneveld SA, Bos AF. Neonatal stress, health, and development in preterms: a systematic review. Pediatr. 2021;148(4):e2021050414. https://doi.org/10.1542/peds.2021-050414.

94. Zhao T, Griffith T, Zhang Y, Li H, Hussain N, Lester B, et al. Early-life factors associated with neurobehavioral outcomes in preterm infants during NICU hospitalization. Pediatr Res. 2022;92(6):1695–704. https://doi.org/10.1038/s41390-022-02021-y.

95. Ullsten A, Campbell-Yeo M, Eriksson M. Parent-led neonatal pain management-a narrative review and update of research and practices. Front Pain Res (Lausanne). 2024;5:1375868. https://doi.org/10.3389/fpain.2024.1375868.

96. Shiff I, Bucsea O, Pillai RR. Psychosocial and neurobiological vulnerabilities of the hospitalized preterm infant and relevant non-pharmacological pain mitigation strategies. Front Pediatr. 2021;9:568755. https://doi.org/10.3389/fped.2021.568755.

97. Sharma N, Samuel AJ. A systematic review of multisensory stimulation on procedural pain among preterm neonates. Pediatr Phys Ther. 2023;35(3):286–91. https://doi.org/10.1097/PEP.0000000000001012.

98. Weng Y, Zhang J, Chen Z. Effect of non-pharmacological interventions on pain in preterm infants in the neonatal intensive care unit: a network meta-analysis of randomized controlled trials. BMC Pediatr. 2024;24:9. https://doi.org/10.1186/s12887-023-04488-y.

99. Pineda R, Kellner P, Guth R, Gronemeyer A, Smith J. NICU sensory experiences associated with positive outcomes: an integrative review of evidence from 2015-2020. J Perinatol. 2023;43(7):837–48. https://doi.org/10.1038/s41372-023-01655-y.

100. Badiee Z, Asghari M, Mohammadizadeh M. The calming effect of maternal breast milk odor on premature infants. Pediatr Neonatol. 2013;54:322–5. https://doi.org/10.1016/j.pedneo.2013.04.004.

101. Sakonidou S, Kotzamanis S, Tallett A, Poots AJ, Modi N, Bell D, et al. Parents' experiences of communication in neonatal care (PEC): a neonatal survey refined for real-time parent feedback. Arch Dis Child Fetal Neonat Ed. 2023;108(4):F416–20. https://doi.org/10.1136/archdischild-2022-324548.

102. Gallagher K, Shaw C, Aladangady N, Marlow N. Parental experience of interaction with healthcare professionals during their infant's stay in the neonatal intensive care unit. Arch Dis Child Fetal Neonat Ed. 2018;103(4):F343–8. https://doi.org/10.1136/archdischild-2016-312278.

103. European Foundation for the Care of newborn infants (EFCNI). Infant and family-centered developmental care. European standards of care for newborn health. Munich: EFCNI; 2018. https://newborn-health-standards.org/downloads/. Accessed 12 August 2024.

104. Fenwick J, Barclay L, Schmied V. 'Chatting': an important clinical tool in facilitating mothering in neonatal nurseries. J Adv Nurs. 2001;33(5):583–93.

105. Petty J, Jarvis J, Thomas R. Listening to the parent voice to inform person-centred neonatal care. J Neonat Nurs. 2019;25(3):121–6. https://doi.org/10.1016/j.jnn.2019.01.005.

106. Voulgaridou A, Paliouras D, Deftereos S, Skarentzos K, Tsergoula E, Miltsakaki I, et al. Hospitalization in neonatal intensive care unit: parental anxiety and satisfaction. Pan Afr Med J. 2023;44:55. https://doi.org/10.11604/pamj.2023.44.55.34344.
107. Schecter R, Pham T, Hua A, Spinazzola R, Sonnenklar J, Li D, et al. Prevalence and longevity of PTSD symptoms among parents of NICU infants analyzed across gestational age categories. Clin Pediatr (Phila). 2020;59(2):163–9. https://doi.org/10.1177/0009922819892046.
108. British Association of Perinatal Medicine, (BAPM). Enhancing shared decision making in neonatal care: a BAPM framework for practice. London: BAPM; 2019.

Specialist Vascular Access Devices

7

Chapter Learning Objectives

Upon completing this chapter, readers will be able to:

- Differentiate clinical situations when specialist vascular access device use is appropriate
  - Specifically: Umbilical venous catheter (UVC), umbilical arterial catheter (UAC), intraosseous (IO) device, intra-arterial catheter (IAC).
- Relate clinical practice strategies for ensuring safe insertion of these specialist devices and routes.
- Apply evidence-based strategies to minimise complications associated with UVC and UAC, such as infection, thrombosis, and catheter migration.
- Critically reflect on how family engagement interventions could be applied during specialist vascular access related procedures.

7.1   Introduction

Vascular access is an almost universal experience for infants in neonatal intensive care units (NICU). The primary routes are by means of peripheral or central venous devices (e.g., PVAD, CVAD, considered in Chaps. 4, 5, and 6). However, other routes are available, and these include intra-arterial catheters (IACs) and intraosseous (IO) devices [1, 2]. In addition, newborn infants provide an opportunity to use the umbilical blood vessels in the devitalised cord stump to obtain vascular access, specifically using umbilical venous (UVC) and arterial (UAC) catheters [3–6]. These specialist devices play an important role in delivering therapies and monitoring vital signs particularly during critical illness or life-threatening situations. This chapter focuses on the insertion, securement, and care of these devices with an emphasis on UVC and UACs. This attention reflects nurses' greater experience and involvement in using these devices in most NICUs. Preventing, identifying, and

© The Author(s), under exclusive license to Springer Nature
Switzerland AG 2024
M. R. van Rens, K. Hugill, *Vascular Access in Neonatal Nursing Practice:
A Neuroprotective Approach*, https://doi.org/10.1007/978-3-031-81602-4_7

limiting the effects of the potentially serious risks associated with using umbilical catheters, IACs, and IO devices is explored.

Pre-procedural skin cleansing and disinfection follows standard practices (see Chaps. 4 and 6). For all catheters placed in the central circulation Surgical-ANTT® should be followed. For all others Standard-ANTT® or Surgical-ANTT® should be followed depending on infant and procedure risk assessment. When asked, adults say that arterial vascular access is more painful than peripheral vein cannulation. It is likely the same for infants and efforts should be made using the range of non-pharmacological and pharmacological pain-relieving and comfort promotion measures used in other areas of vascular access (see Chaps. 4 and 6). For example, non-nutritive sucking, sucrose solutions/breastmilk, and swaddling can be helpful and provide opportunities for parents to play an active role and reduce infant stress and promote quicker post-procedure recovery [1–3]. Whilst topical anaesthetic agents (e.g., EMLA®) are largely discounted in neonatal practice due to concern about unpredictable skin absorption, their use can nullify the initial pain associated with arterial puncture and reduce reactive vasospasm making the procedure easier.

7.2   Umbilical Vascular Catheters

In newborn infants within the first few days of life, it is possible to utilise the devitalised umbilical vein and arteries to obtain central vascular access [2, 3, 6]. This unique situation confers advantages and additional hazards. Experts state that umbilical catheterisation is a viable option for infants who are less than 2 days old [3–5, 7–9]. Decisions to insert an umbilical catheter should be based upon considerations of the severity of presenting illness (e.g., severe newborn respiratory distress (NRDS) or therapeutic hypothermia) and the availability of other routes for vascular access [3, 5].

7.2.1   Umbilical Vein Catheters (UVC)

UVCs made from polyurethane (PUR) are widely used in NICUs for short duration vascular access in the immediate post-birth period. These devices are suitable for preterm infants and those with haemodynamic instability or affected by serious neonatal disorders (e.g., hypoxia) [4–6]. In practice, UVCs can be especially helpful in securing vascular access amongst extremely preterm infants during the first few days when peripheral access can be more difficult to obtain due to oedema.

Catheters should be removed and replaced with alternative vascular access as soon as practicable as this significantly reduces infection risk. However, the exact timing of removal is uncertain with timelines between 4 and 7 days recommended [3–5, 9, 10]. Longer dwell times for UVCs in infants with severe skin conditions or those without alternative vascular access can be considered after careful review of the risks and benefits of doing this, but these will be on a case-by-case basis. Whilst UVCs offer specific benefits, UACs serve as an alternative essential route for monitoring and therapy.

7.2.2 Umbilical Arterial Catheters (UAC)

Many NICUs guidelines restrict the use of UACs to a limited range of situations to reduce the risks associated with their use [5]. Indications for UAC insertion include the need for frequent blood sampling, continuous blood pressure, or blood gas monitoring. This might need a reference. Although many NICUs avoid infusing medications through UACs due to the risks of vasospasm, thromboembolism, and arterial injury, some studies report limited use of UACs for parenteral nutrition and fluids in emergency situations. Current guidelines emphasise avoiding vasoactive drugs and calcium boluses. A review by Ullman et al. [6] on catheter safety stresses that, whenever possible, alternative routes such as central venous access should be used to avoid arterial complications. Contraindications for umbilical catheterisation are few but include:

- Congenital abdominal wall defects
- Abnormal cord blood vessels
- Infant age beyond 2 days
- Localised infection around the cord stump
- Sepsis

7.2.2.1 UAC and UVC Insertion

Umbilical vein and artery catheterisation differs from most approaches to vascular access in that the blood vessels are readily accessible through the cord stump and venipuncture, or arterial puncture is not required. Insertion, in some respects is largely unchanged from the early days of neonatology [3, 5]. Challenges include catheter navigation, tip confirmation, avoidance of creating false passages or aneurisms, and deciding how best to secure the catheter to prevent catheter migration [3, 5, 11–15]. Numerous instructional materials are readily available in the public domain and highlight the commonalities and features of different healthcare providers' technique (e.g., [3, 16, 17]).

Real-time ultrasound-guidance is increasingly recognised as the gold standard for UVC and UAC insertion, significantly reducing the incidence of malposition and vascular injury. A study by Seigel et al. [13] showed that ultrasound-guided insertion led to a reduction in complications, particularly in extremely preterm neonates, where anatomical landmarks are less reliable. Post-insertion, it is essential to verify the catheter tip position to avoid error, this should also be conducted using ultrasound rather than relying solely on X-rays (Text Box 7.1).

Text Box 7.1 Practice Point: Overcoming Resistance During Umbilical Catheter Insertion
Sometimes as the catheter exits the cord and enters the body through the umbilical ring, an increase in resistance can be felt.

- It is important not to overapply pressure as this can lead to blood vessel rupture (especially umbilical vein) and the creation of a false passage, resulting in a failed insertion attempt.
  - Gentle traction on the cord directed towards the lower abdomen can help the catheter navigate this point and its entry into the internal vasculature, confirmed by the ability to aspirate blood.

Several different methods to estimate catheter insertion length are described (e.g., [3, 5]). Most estimations use a combination of infant weight or external anatomical measurements as a predicative tool. One example uses shoulder to umbilicus distance and reference nomographs to determine catheter length [5]. Regardless of which calculation is used, all have margins of error that can lead to suboptimal catheter tip location. Real-time ultrasound-guided umbilical catheter insertion offers promise to eradicate the need for these calculations and post-procedural radiological confirmation of tip position (5, 12, 14, 18–20).

Small variations in the depth of insertion can result in significant malposition. Traditional methods to help determine catheter length to achieve the desired tip location involved experience-based approaches, predictive estimates based on anatomical measurements, and later confirmation using X-radiography images viewed against anatomical landmarks, particularly vertebral [1, 3, 5, 12, 21]. This approach is considered inaccurate [12], and newer predictive modelling tools such as the 'UmbiCalc mobile application' have been proposed to update these traditional methods [21] (Text Box 7.2).

Text Box 7.2: Practice Point: Distinguishing a UVC from a UAC on Radiograph
On radiography, UVCs can be distinguished from UVCs by their routing.

- UVCs travel directly upwards (cranially).
- UACs initially travels downwards (caudally) before reaching a common iliac vessel and ascending cranially.

7.2.2.2 UVC Tip Position

For a UVC, the ideal catheter tip position is anatomically located between vertebrae T8 and T9, that is, above the liver but below the heart [3, 5]. Catheter tips located above T8 or in the heart are too high and in this situation the catheter should be partially withdrawn. Catheter tips situated below T10-L1 should be used cautiously and replaced as soon as possible as catheters in this location carry higher risks of complication [3, 5, 22]. Any catheter that is in the liver or follows an uncertain or tortuous path should be removed and not used. One exception to this guidance is the use of UVCs during stabilisation and resuscitation when the catheter is often inserted using experience. If used during emergencies, then the catheter should only be inserted a few centimetres beyond the abdominal wall to avoid potential misdirection into the liver and harm arising from bolus fluid injections [1–3].

7.2.2.3 UAC Tip Position

The usual navigation of a UAC is that after passing through the cord stump and umbilical ring it enters the common iliac artery and then progresses to the aorta. In practice, the catheter tip can be safely located in one of the two locations. Optimally, the catheter tip should be in a 'high' position anatomically located between T6 and T10 vertebrae. Alternatively, in some clinical circumstances a 'low' position at L3 to L5 and below the major aortic branches can be acceptable for short durations. However, intermediate positions are undesirable due to the potential for occlusion of other blood vessels by the catheter.

Unfortunately, recent studies indicate that confirmation of catheter tip position through radiological images may be imprecise [12, 19, 20]. Rubortone et al. [20] mapped radiographs against ultrasound confirmed correct tip position for UVCs. Most were located around T8 or T9, but there were outlier patients that had their tips appearing to be located at T7 and T10 despite ultrasound confirmation of correct tip position. This means that healthcare providers relying on radiology alone might have incorrectly interpreted catheter tip positions as either too shallow or too deep and acted accordingly, which might not have been in the infant's best interest.

7.2.2.4 Securement and Dressing

Choices around CVAD securement and dressing affect catheter performance and complication risks. Whilst the principles for fixation and stabilisation are generally similar, there are distinct considerations for UVCs and UACs. Securing umbilical catheters presents unique problems due to their positioning and remnants of the cord stump. This makes catheter dislodgement or accidental removal during patient handling a greater concern than with other CVADs [14]. There are different approaches to securement, and, currently, there is limited consensus about which is the superior method. Older approaches used a variety of vertical and horizontal non-sterile tapes secured to the cord stump, catheter, and skin to create a supporting framework. These designs were variously termed 'goalposts', 'anchors', or 'bridges' depending on local idiom. Now, it is common to use sutures secured through the cord stump and then wound around the catheter [3], with or without additional tape to contain the sutures. This approach avoids direct application of medical adhesives to the skin and enables any remaining cord stump to naturally desiccate. However, it does leave open the possibility of extraluminal microbial contamination.

Recent study has demonstrated the efficacy of using cyanoacrylate tissue adhesive as an adjunct to suture-based securement for UVCs. One randomised controlled trial ($n = 130$) compared sutures and sutures with adjunct cyanoacrylate surgical glue (Gluban 2® (GEM srl)) [14]. Catheter dislodgment in the first 48 h after insertion was significantly lower in the suture and applied adhesive group (1.5% versus

23.1%, $P < 0.01$). Measured over the whole dwell time, this relationship was sustained (7.7% versus 24.6%, $P = 0.16$). Other measures, including infection and thrombosis did not achieve statistical significance.

After 72–96 h, tissue adhesive seemed less effective at limiting catheter movement [14]. This finding might be related to natural breakdown of adhesive bonding of biodegradation of the glue. Gluban 2 is formulated as a biodegradable N-butyl-cyanoacrylate base with an attached monomer (methacryloxysulfone). The product is CE and FDA approved for surgical vascular closure and endovascular use in neuronal radiology but not for use in vascular access. The benefits reported from using cyanoacrylate tissue adhesive for catheter securement seem transferable to umbilical catheters. However, further study using formulations specific for vascular access is required.

One alternative engineered umbilical catheter securement aid is the LifeBubble™ (Laborie Medical Technologies). This device, made from silicone designed into a raised three-dimensional clamp like fastening allows for air flow around the still visible cord stump. It is secured to the skin with bespoke hydrocolloid tapes and can secure up to two catheters. In one small study (n = 118), this device performed better than the comparator (sterile tapes secured to skin) at preventing catheter tip migration [15]. When they become available, results from studies comparing this device with more robust securement approaches will likely inform debates about optimal umbilical catheter securement.

Exit site (i.e., cord stump) dressing is contentious. The current cord care paradigm advocates maintaining a dry umbilical cord to facilitate speedier separation of the devitalised cord stump. After umbilical catheterisation, some maintain this stance either overtly or by implication. In contrast, others advocate that the umbilical catheters be treated like any other CVAD, and the exit site dressed (see Chap. 6). Proponents of dressing cite on balance a greater risk of extraluminal contamination and infection and that the usual short dwell time of most UVC and UACs is unlikely to unduly affect natural cord separation.

Because of concerns about clinical instability, accidental removal, or dislodgment, there is sometimes hesitancy amongst parents and nurses over infant handling. However, with effective securement and dressing, this concern should not limit opportunities for physical parent–infant contact when critical illness resolves. It might be that exit site dressing could enable greater parent–infant contact by subliminally signalling that UVC and UACs should be treated in the same way as other CVADs. However, in the absence of definite evidence, nurses should adhere to institutional guidelines for catheter securement and exit site care.

7.2.2.5 Complications Associated with Umbilical Catheters

Umbilical catheters are well tolerated by most infants, but complications can occur. For UVCs, concerns centre around the effects of malposition and catheter tip migration [3, 5, 8–12, 19, 22–25]. UVC tip migration can occur independently of catheter dislodgment. Clinicians have observed that UVC tip migration occurs frequently, especially with longer dwell times [19, 20]. Exact explanation for this phenomenon is unclear. It might be related to initial insertion length, body positional changes, or variations in abdominal pressure, for example [12, 20]. The use of serial bedside ultrasound to monitor for thrombus formation or tip migration is critical. A systematic review by Gibson et al. [24] emphasised that repeated imaging throughout the catheter's dwell time can significantly reduce the risk of severe complications such as thrombosis and infection. Proactive removal or replacement of the catheter should occur upon any signs of migration or thrombus formation.

For UACs, severe vasospasm and micro-thromboembolic complications resulting in tissue ischaemia and necrosis rank highly amongst healthcare provider concerns [24]. Table 7.1 lists reported complications associated with umbilical catheterisation.

Table 7.1 Complications associated with umbilical catheterisation

Complication	Reported in connection to UVC	Reported in connection to UAC
Accidental artery perforation (false aneurism)		✓
Cardiac tamponade	✓	
Vein perforation (false lumens)	✓	
Inadvertent umbilical artery cannulation	✓	
Catheter misdirection into liver	✓	
Hepatic damage (abscess, necrosis)	✓	
Portal vein thrombosis	✓	
Cardiac arrhythmia	✓	
Pleural effusion	✓	
Infection (localised and bloodstream)	✓	✓
Catheter dislodgement	✓	✓
Air embolism	✓	✓
Thrombosis	✓	✓
Bleeding at insertion site (cord)	✓	✓
Catheter tip migration	✓	✓
Vasospasm		✓
Discoloration of toes		✓
Blanching of leg or buttocks		✓
Limb ischemia		✓
Occlusion of major blood vessels (malposition)		✓
Necrotising enterocolitis (with prolonged dwell time)	✓	✓
Catheter occlusion	✓	✓

7.3   Intra-Arterial Catheters (IAC)

In addition to the umbilical arteries, there are several other potential sites for arterial catheter insertion in NICU infants. These sites include the peripheral and major arteries of the upper and lower limbs and the temporal artery [1, 26–31].

7.3.1   Upper Limb IAC

In the upper limbs, these include the brachial, radial, and ulnar arteries in the wrist and supplying the hand and arm. The radial and ulnar arteries are subsidiaries of the brachial artery higher up the arm and are intimately interconnected. Connected networks of blood vessels from these two arteries create a collateral circulation known as the superior and inferior palmar arch. Figure 7.1 shows a simplified diagrammatic representation. Cadaver and surgical studies point out that between 20% and 30% of people have anatomical variants of this arrangement [32, 33]. This can have implications when considering IAC insertion. Consequently, it is essential before accessing these arteries to confirm the presence of functional collateral circulation to avoid potential ischaemia should one artery become occluded.

7.3.2   Lower Limb IAC

Like in the wrist and hand, several arteries contribute to anastomotic networks to provide a collateral blood supply to the foot and ankle. These arteries include the dorsalis pedis and posterior and anterior tibial arteries which give rise to interconnected networks, including the arcuate artery on the dorsum of the foot and the plantar arch on the sole of the foot. Also in the lower limb is the major femoral artery accessible in the groin, which supplies the legs through continuity with the popliteal and anterior and posterior tibial arteries and collateral blood vessels.

In neonates, excluding UACs the radial artery is the most commonly used site for an IAC, representing around 63% of insertions [28], followed by the posterior tibia. The dorsalis pedis arteries feature less frequently in reports, perhaps reflecting technical issues with avoiding occlusion due to flexion. In practice, some advocate avoiding the brachial and femoral arteries as the consequences from losing blood supply are too great. In the past, the ulnar site was largely excluded as it was considered less favourable due to technical difficulties in accessing. However, with the greater use of imaging technologies, this situation is likely to change (Text Box 7.3).

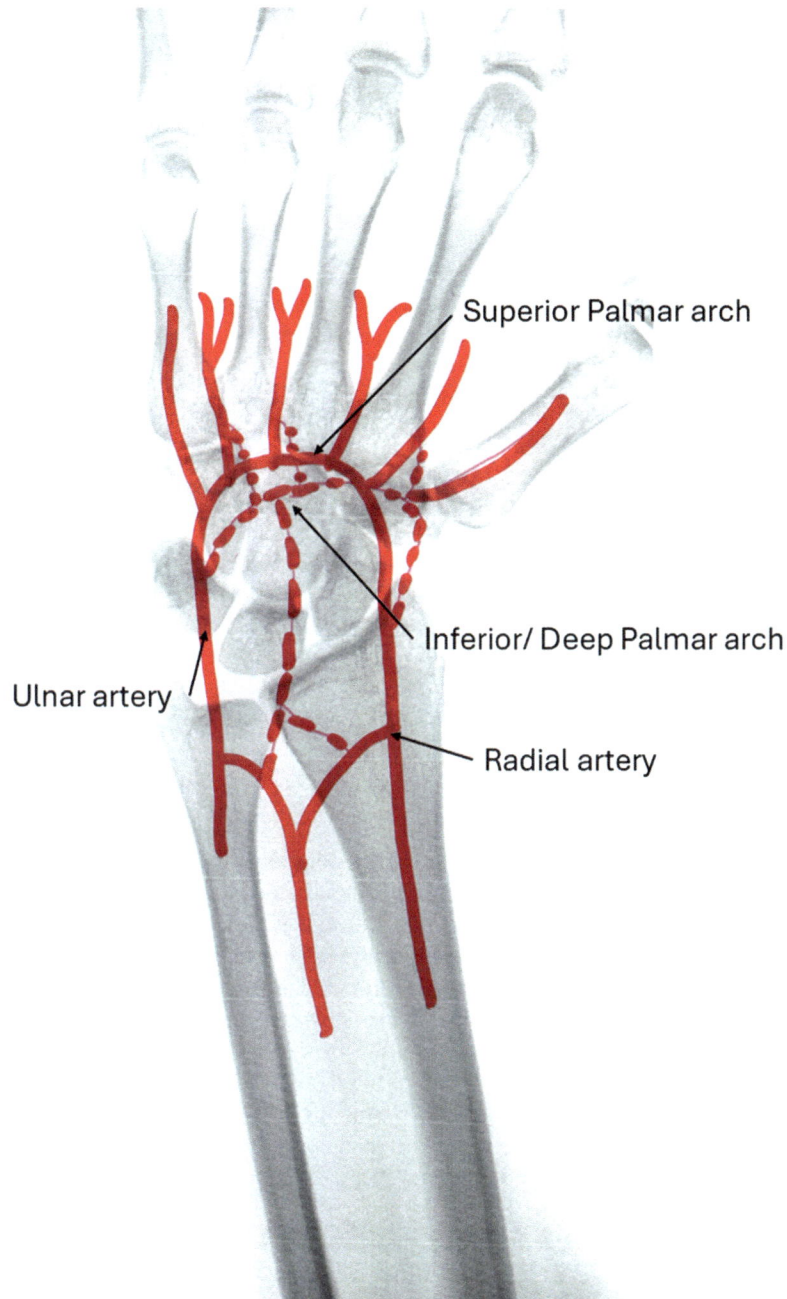

Fig. 7.1 Diagrammatic representation of the palmar arches of the hand

Text Box 7.3 Practice Point: Allen Test

A simple bedside assessment of the adequacy of collateral circulation in the hand by assessing the patency of the radial and ulnar arteries.

How to conduct the Allen test, modified for infants.

1. Preparation, explain to the infant's parents present why you are doing the test and what is involved. Position the infant comfortably with their arm positioned at the level of the heart. Test the left and right hand separately, allowing enough time for infant recovery between tests.
2. Palpation, identify and gently palpate the radial and ulnar arteries at the wrist.
3. Occlusion, apply pressure to both the radial and ulnar arteries simultaneously, effectively occluding both. This temporarily stops blood flow to the hand.
4. Release, whilst maintaining pressure on both arteries have an assistant or parent, gently form a fist with the infant's hand, repeat several times.
5. Release pressure on the ulnar artery whilst still occluding the radial artery and the infant's hand is formed in a fist.
6. Observe the infant's palm and fingers. If the ulnar artery provides adequate collateral circulation, the patient's palm and fingers should regain their normal colour within a few seconds.
7. Repeat steps 3–6, releasing pressure on the radial artery and document your findings in the infant's electronic health record and n-VAMP.

The purpose of doing the Allen test is to help determine if there is sufficient collateral blood flow from the ulnar artery to the hand. This is in case the radial artery is temporarily or permanently compromised during IAC insertion and use. It is important to note that whilst this test provides valuable information about collateral circulation in the hand, its predictive value for avoiding ischemic complications is limited. The test is a subjective qualitative assessment and may not provide precise measurements of blood flow. In most cases, it is considered advisable to conduct further comprehensive assessments using ultrasound [34–37].

Mavarez et al. [34] carried out an ultrasound evaluation of internal radial artery diameter in 50 infants aged between birth and six-months of age. Ultrasound measurement of radial artery C:V ratios (see Chap. 6) found that a 22 G cannula created 100% occlusion of the artery lumen and using a 24 G device occlusion was between 75% and 99%. Given concern over the impacts on venous circulation and complications from adverse C:V ratios about 33% (see Chap. 6, Sect. 6.3.2), this finding is problematic. One study, involving adult patients reported that locating the point of catheter insertion away from areas of flexion combined with pre-procedural ultrasound assessment of vessel suitability was associated with increased functional dwell time [39]. It is likely that situating IACs away from points of flexion might archive similar effects though in practice doing this can be difficult.

7.3.3 IAC Insertion, Securement, and Removal

The insertion of IACs into peripheral arteries can often involve using a direct method like PVAD insertion though with adjustment to the angle of insertion to account for the deeper location of arteries compared to peripheral veins. Some healthcare providers preferentially opt for catheters made from PUR material, though without a stylet (mandarin) these can kink during arterial catheterisation [27, 28, 30]. In contrast others prefer materials like PEBA. Whilst, catheters made from PEBA are resistant to collapse the inherent stiffness of this material can also be problematic for unfamiliar users. The addition of a stylet (mandarin) to the insertion kit can prevent thrombus formation during cannulation of the artery, some device designs incorporate non-return valves with the same objective to prevent backflow. Alternatively, for deeper located and major arteries, the Seldinger technique is preferred [38], ideally accompanied by ultrasound guidance [35–37, 40].

IACs require stable securement but rigorous comparative evidence about how best to do this is uncertain and further research is necessary to determine optimal strategies [41]. Current methods include a combination of standard or bordered dressing, sutureless devices, and integrated devices. The role of cyanoacrylate tissue adhesive for IAC securement is largely unexplored. However, research into the use of tissue adhesives for adjunct securement and exit site sealing during extracorporeal membrane oxygenation is supportive [42]. In practice, some NICUs have extended its use based on data from CVAD, UVC, and PVAD research. In the absence of definitive evidence, nurses should follow local advice until such time more robust evidence becomes available.

The removal of any IAC requires a considered and systematic approach to ensure patient safety. Most units using IACs have guidelines setting out specific steps. These can include advice around the timing during the day for removal, the presence of key healthcare providers, attention to aseptic technique, infant positioning, pain relief, and comfort measures. In addition, these guidelines often contain explicit instruction on ensuring patient saftey during and after removal. For example, how to remove dressings or securement aids, how speedily to withdraw the catheter, how long to apply pressure post-removal to control bleeding, and post procedure exit site observation.

7.3.4 Complications Associated with IAC

The primary concerns about complications associated with IAC relate to those around insertion and the effects of impaired blood flow due to reversible or irreversible arterial occlusion. Following femoral artery IAC one study [31] reported post-removal loss of pedal pulse or bilateral discrepancies. In this study, there was an association between the loss of pedal pulse and larger catheters (>2.5 Fr). Synnes and colleagues [43] presented two case studies of limb shortening due to growth plate arrest and an association with IAC use. On investigation, the shared common features in the two cases were preterm birth and the use of a femoral arterial line on

Table 7.2 Complications
associated with IAC
insertion and use

Pain
Air embolism
Vasospasm
Bleeding trauma to artery
Thrombosis and micro-emboli formation leading to blood vessel and/or catheter occlusion
Haematoma formation
Nerve damage
Temporary impairment of peripheral circulation
Skin colour changes
Skin blanching
Limb ischaemia
Limb growth plate arrest—Later limb shortening
Loss or alterations in pedal pulse
Unredeemable ischaemia
Tissue necrosis
Digit, hand, leg amputation

the same side of the body as the shortened limb. These findings imply potential real-world effects from partial arterial lumen occlusion due to IAC presence and reinforce the need for detailed pre-procedural assessment of vessel suitability [34]. Table 7.2 summarises reported complications [28–31, 43–51].

Many complications associated with IACs can be avoided by judicious precautions during pre-procedural assessment and insertion. However, vasospasm and impaired peripheral perfusion and ischaemia remain problematic. Generally, catheter removal can resolve these problems [45], but on occasion ischaemia is persistent risking tissue necrosis and the continued viability of digits and whole limbs. The level of intervention is determined by extent of tissue involvement and can include conservative measures, application of topical vasorelaxants, anticoagulant thrombolysis, nerve block, and surgery. Primary standard non-invasive interventions include catheter removal, limb elevation, and warming of contra lateral extremity to induce reflexive vasodilation secondary. Early consultation with the vascular team is advisable.

There are several reports of successfully using 2% topical glycerine trinitrate (GTN) formulations to relieve peripheral ischaemia by promoting vascular relaxation [46–48]. Evidence for the effectiveness of GTN is mainly limited to positive case reports [48]. However, this situation might reflect a reporting and publication bias for 'good news'. Some commentators advocate caution in this approach as there is a risk of unpredictable absorption and possible wider systemic effects beyond the target area and theoretical evidence that GTN might affect cerebral blood flow [48]. Currently, there are no unified guidelines regarding best formulation, dose, frequency, or duration of treatment for GTN, and more detailed studies of biological mechanism and clinical utility are required [49].

In neonates, there is high frequency of bleeding complications associated with fibrinolytic and anticoagulant therapy for limb ischaemia due to thrombosis [50]. Concern over side effects often precludes the use of these therapies [50].

Case reports regarding the successful use of peripheral nerve block can reduce vascular spasm and relieve the effects of thrombosis [50, 51]. However, there are currently no comparative studies to determine the generalisability of this approach in neonatal settings. Most complications associated with IACs are transient and resolved by catheter removal though others can be devastating and life altering. Taking measures to avoid the occurrence of complications would seem the optimal strategy.

7.4   Intraosseous (IO) Access to the Circulation

Emergency vascular access is rarely required during neonatal resuscitation, but when it is required, the umbilical vein is the preferred route to provide medications or fluids [2]. However, if the umbilical route is not available, intraosseous (IO) access is feasible as an emergency measure [2, 52–54]. Mileder et al. [55] surveyed 5 years data about IO use during neonatal resuscitation. They reported that IO was only rarely attempted during neonatal resuscitation. This finding might be partly attributable accounted for the observation in practice that emergency vascular access is seldom required neonatal resuscitation; the focus being on managing the airway and supporting transitions to breathing generally been sufficient.

The technique varies slightly depending on the IO device and whether manual insertion or mechanical drilling is used. IO insertion involves penetrating the outer cortex of a long bone to access the inner medullary cavity, which is connected to the systemic circulation. As the medullary cavity is essentially non-collapsable, doing this can provide direct vascular access when shock or venous collapse prevents more usual routes of access [52, 56]. In neonates, the preferred site for IO device insertion is the tibial bone as other potential sites used in older children and adults lack the necessary medullar space to be safely used [57–59]. The list of contraindications is few but includes:

- Fracture in the target bone
- Congenital disorders of bone development
- Previous failed attempts in the same bone site
- Lack of available competent healthcare provider

With training, IOs can be readily placed in neonates for the administration of volume expanding fluids and adrenaline during resuscitation, but there is a small margin for error in neonates compared to older children [56].

7.4.1   Complications Associated with IO Devices

The IO route can be lifesaving when other options are not available [60], but the range of severity of potential complications is worrying [56, 60–64]. However, most are rare though some mild effects are reported in around 30% of survivors [61]. Schwindt et al. [53] provide some insights into the use, effectiveness, and complications from using IO during stabilisation of critical ill infants. This review of 2 years of surveillance data from German hospitals identified 161 occasions when IO was

Table 7.3 Complications associated with intraosseous (IO) access

Failure to insert
Inadvertent penetration of the distal cortex of the bone
Bent or broken IO needle
Needle occlusion with bone marrow or thrombi
Tibial fracture
Needle dislodgment
Local swelling around insertion site
Haematoma
Infiltration of fluid—Subperiosteal, subcutaneous
Poor healing
Soft tissue infection
Osteomyelitis
Post-insertion perfusion issues—compartment syndrome
Necrosis—Skin, soft tissue, and bone
Amputation
Growth plate arrest—Subsequent limb shortening
Pain

attempted during infant stabilisation. 146 devices were successfully inserted from 206 attempts. Over half of these infants (64%, n = 103) survived to discharge. Most successful insertions were in the proximal tibia and were left in place for under 3 minutes. Complications recorded included minor swelling and misplaced devices. In nine cases (6%), major complications including broken IO needle, soft tissue damage, necrosis peripheral perfusion compromise and osteomyelitis occurred [53]. Table 7.3 summarises the major complications associated with IO access and Text Box 7.4 draws attention to one rare condition reportedly associated with IO use.

Text Box 7.4 Practice Point: Compartment Syndrome

Compartment syndrome arises due to increased pressure in enclosed spaces. This can restrict localised blood flow causing ischaemia and impaired cellular gas exchange leading to pallor and reduced pulse in affected areas and tissue necrosis. Report from adults highlights the condition is accompanied by intense pain.

The condition though rare in infants has been reported in connection with IO and umbilical catheters; it can present as a surgical emergency requiring prompt relief of pressure by fasciotomy.

In essence, IO access might be appropriate in neonatal emergencies when more usual vascular access is not available. However, there is limited evidence to guide practice about the optimal choice of IO device, insertion site, insertion technique (operator pressure or power driver), dwell time, and further research is required.

7.5   Vascular Access in Specialist Situations

Vascular access is sometimes required for specialist applications. Examples include cardiac catheterisation for investigative or therapeutic interventions, haemodialysis, or exchange blood transfusion. Some of these like haemodialysis are currently rare in NICUs, though this situation might change in the future [65–68]. Exchange transfusion, used for the treatment of hyperbilirubinemia and haemolytic disease of the foetus and newborn (HDFN) is now less commonly seen in practice. In many countries, this decline is attributable to preventative strategies (e.g. RhD immunisation, intrauterine transfusions) and the availability of less invasive and effective treatments for reducing bilirubin levels [69–71]. Advances in non-invasive imaging technologies such as 3D scanning and printing have seen a decline in the use of cardiac catheterisation for diagnostic purposes [72, 73].

Considered together, many of these specialist vascular access situations face similar changes in practice. Establishing an infrastructure and maintaining skilled teams to support these approaches is expensive. Health economics and calculations of benefit, risk, and cost will factor into decisions about their obtainability, whilst technical challenges familiar to other fields of neonatal vascular access also feature. For example, ensuring haemodynamic and physiological stability in often critically ill infants during use, the design and sourcing of catheters small enough for neonatal vasculatures and yet capable of therapeutic use, and the avoidance of major known complications.

7.5.1   Advanced Extracorporeal Life Support

Advanced extracorporeal life support (ECLS) technology and its synonymous term ECMO (extracorporeal membrane oxygenation) were first successfully used with neonates in the 1970s [74]. However, it remains a niche subspecialty within neonatal care [74]. This therapy requires specific infrastructure, multidisciplinary teamworking, and healthcare provider knowledge and clinical expertise to manage the presenting condition and post-birth physiology whilst delivering treatment safely. Detailed consideration of the use of ECLS in neonates is beyond the scope of this book, but for readers interested in gaining additional insight into this topic should access links to further reading and training (e.g., [74–78], https://www.elso.org).

Generally, in neonates, ECLS is used for conditions with impaired gas exchange due to reversible or treatable cardio-pulmonary dysfunction. Amongst neonatal ECLS patients around 75% of them have conditions of impaired gaseous exchange, specifically, meconium aspiration syndrome (MAS), or congenital diaphragmatic hernia (CDH), or persistent pulmonary hypertension of the newborn (PPHN). The remaining 25% of patients have congenital heart disorders [74, 79].

Research and registry reports (e.g., [80], https://elso.org) indicate around 84% treatment survival and between 50 and 97% (overall 73%) survival to discharge amongst all neonates receiving ECLS [80]. However, these figures might reflect highly selective patient referral protocols and mask variations between centres. Some of this variation relates to underlying primary diagnosis, infants with reversible respiratory conditions tend to have greater survival than those with congenital cardiac conditions requiring surgery, for example. Long-term monitoring of morbidities associated with ECLS reflects concerns about potentially adverse neurodevelopment due to cerebral bleeds and the effects of potentially comprised cerebral blood flow after cannula removal. Data to date suggest that whilst neurological deficits occur, their incidence and severity are comparable to that seen in similar groups of infants treated more conventionally [79, 80].

Vascular access is often gained through surgical cannulation of the internal jugular vein or common carotid artery using the Seldinger technique, increasingly with real-time ultrasound guidance (see Chap. 6). Femoral blood vessels are rarely used in infants and pre-walking children as they lack capacity to accommodate the required flow rates [74–76, 81–83]. The choice of using double lumen veno-venous or veno-arterial cannula is dictated by clinical need and the availability of suitable vessels [84, 85]. V-V routes are primarily aimed at delivering pulmonary support and VA routes are more effective at providing cardiorespiratory support. Cannula size, the diameter of central blood vessels, and how easily they can be dilated are major limitations when determining which patients can have the therapy [84, 85].

Until recently, ECLS was restricted to larger and more mature infants due to concerns about cerebral haemorrhage related to anticoagulant use within ECLS delivery circuits and the physical size of blood vessels to accommodate the cannula. Small (<2 kg) and preterm infants (<34 weeks gestation) were contraindications for ECLS. Some centres have reported successful therapy in infants of less than 2 kg and below 34 weeks gestational age [86]. This has led to a reframing of absolute and relative contraindications for therapy. Patients below 30 weeks gestation or 1 kg remain absolute contraindications, but those who are above 34 weeks or 2 kg could be considered as relative contraindicated for ECLS. However, when ECLS is used for smaller and more immature infants, results indicate increased rates of intraventricular haemorrhage and lower survival. Though these risks might be acceptable in some circumstances, the decision to use ECLS should be taken on a case-by-case basis. For high-risk procedures like ECLS with uncertain life-long consequences (e.g., due to potential loss of functioning blood vessel or cerebral haemorrhage), decisions about referral for treatment must take into account the context of the clinical situation, foreseeable response of infant to intervention, and most essentially parents' (informed) wishes.

Most parents encountering the possibility of their infant requiring ECLS will be faced with acute life-threatening illness and having to cope with all additional stresses and emotions that such situations bring about. During difficult conversations about treatment options, informed consent, and survival, there might seem little time to consider less critical topics beyond the immediacy of the current situation. However, this does not mean such topics are less important. Pre-empting negative feelings of loss, shock guilt, depression, hopelessness, emotional disengagement, uncertainty, anger, fear, and isolation that are common amongst parents facing critical events and responding with empathy, kindliness, and compassion can be influential on how bad news is received and managed.

Providing support and guiding parents through practical ways so they can continue to support their infant, such as providing breastmilk, touching, and talking to their infant can rebalance feelings around emotional control. Infants receiving ECLS will often be transferred to other departments or facilities depending on how the service is organised. This can create additional barriers for parental presence and involvement, for example by obliging them to travel long distances to unfamiliar places. Whilst the UN Convention on the Rights of the Child underlines the right of children to be close to their parents [87]. Ensuring that this happens during specialist treatments is challenging, but providing financial support or transport, and onsite parent and family accommodation can be helpful if universally available.

7.6   Concluding Remarks

Specialist vascular access devices such as those considered in this chapter form an important element of the neonatal vascular access repertoire. Umbilical catheters, particularly UVCs are commonly used in NICUs, but using them is not risk free. Nurses and other healthcare providers need to remain vigilant to prevent complications occurring. IO devices when used in extremis can be lifesaving. To use them safely and efficiently requires training, competence, and the use of strategies to maintain competence. As a rule of thumb, the beneficial effects of IAC insertion should always be balanced by an evaluation of the risk of complications. When using umbilical catheters (UVC, UAC) and IACs catheter tip verification, and surveillance combined with effective catheter securement are key to ensuring safe optimal use. Evidence to date supports the view that ultrasound is the best modality for the accurate confirmation of UVC, UAC, and IAC catheter tip position. However, further research into best practices for catheter insertion, securement, and complication management is required to enhance neonatal outcomes.

Key Points
- Umbilical catheters and IACs provide an important option for vascular access in neonates.
- IO devices can be safely used to secure vascular access in emergencies when other routes are not available.
- Surgical-ANTT® is mandatory during central vascular catheter insertion (UVC/UAC, femoral IAC), the only exception is during umbilical catheterisation in emergency lifesaving situations.
  - For other IACs, the choice of Surgical-ANTT® or Standard-ANTT® approach should be based on an assessment of contamination risk and procedural complexity.

- Neonatal IAC insertion requires nurses and other healthcare providers to have an advanced knowledge of anatomy base and demonstrate considerable dexterity and proficiency in practice.
- Ultrasound-guided insertion and catheter tip confirmation for UVC, UAC, and IAC is feasible and increasingly desirable for safe practice.
- There is uncertainty about how best to secure and dress umbilical and IAC exit sites, and more comparative research is required.
  - There is some evidence that cyanoacrylate tissue adhesive formulations can provide important additional securement and exit site protection for UVC and ECMO cannula; this might be transferable to UAC and IACs.
- Umbilical, IAC and IO devices are associated with a range of serious and life-altering complication.
  - Planned early removal can mitigate complications risks, particularly those associated with infection, thrombosis, and catheter migration.
  - Evidence concerning the efficacy of treatment for ischaemic complications is underdeveloped and requires further study.

Reflective Activity Read the following case related to a complication arising from vascular access and consider your responses to the reflective questions at the end.

Ezra, a 4-day-old preterm infant born at 25 week gestation, has been seriously unstable due to his prematurity and having a congenital infection. He has two vascular access devices in place, a UAC and an n-PICC. The UAC is being used for monitoring his blood pressure and blood sampling. During hygiene care, you notice some slight but obvious blanching of his left buttock, feet, and toes.

You report this to the medical staff present. This person seems unconcerned as the blanching is only 'very mild' and states that the UAC does not need to be removed. They maintain that there is a need to continue using the IAC to obtain blood samples and by doing this it will preserve Ezra's veins and heals from harm and expose him to less pain. They suggest you cover the opposite leg with a blanket to stimulate reflexive vasodilation.

Considering the above case and your reading in this chapter, reflect on your answers to the following questions:

1. Do you agree with this proposed course of action?
   (a) Consider, is the rationale to prevent pain and vascular injury sound reasoning for this course of action, what are the risks from continuing to use the UAC?

2. If you disagree, how will you explain your reasoning for an alternate course of action to your colleague?
   (a) Think about which unit protocols and guidelines might apply and your responsibilities for patient advocacy around preventing harm and pain.
3. Reflect on how might you resolve any disagreement over Ezra's management?
   (a) Think about the need for respectful communication, escalation policies, and documentation.

References

1. Nickel B, Gorski L, Kleidon T, Kyes A, DeVries M, Keogh S, et al. Infusion therapy standards of practice. 9th ed. J Inf Nurs. 2024;47(1S):S1–285. https://doi.org/10.1097/NAN.0000000000000532.
2. Madar J, Roehr CR, Ainsworth S, Ersdal H, Morley C, RÜdiger M, et al. European Resuscitation Council guidelines 2021: newborn resuscitation and support of transition of infants at birth. Resuscitation 2021;161: 291–326. https://doi.org/10.1016/j.resuscitation.2021.02.014.
3. British Association of Perinatal Medicine, (BAPM). Use of central venous catheters in neonates a framework for practice. London: BAPM; 2018.
4. Barone G, D'Andrea V, Ancora G, Cresi F, Maggio L, Capasso A, et al. The neonatal DAV-expert algorithm: a GAVeCeLT/GAVePed consensus for the choice of the most appropriate venous access in newborns. Eur J Pediatr. 2023;182(8):3385–95. https://doi.org/10.1007/s00431-023-04984-4.
5. D'Andrea V, Prontera G, Rubortone SA, Pezza L, Pinna G, Barone G, et al. Umbilical venous catheter update: a narrative review including ultrasound and training. Front Pediatr. 2022;9:774705. https://doi.org/10.3389/fped.2021.774705.
6. Ullman AJ, Bernstein SJ, Brown E, Aiyagari R, Doellman D, Faustino EVS, et al. The Michigan appropriateness guide for intravenous catheters in pediatrics: miniMAGIC. Pediatrics. 2020;145(Suppl 3):S269–84. https://doi.org/10.1542/peds.2019-3474I.
7. Bjorland PA, Øymar K, Ersdal HL, Rettedal SI. Incidence of newborn resuscitative interventions at birth and short-term outcomes: a regional population-based study. BMJ Paediatr Open. 2019;3(1):e000592. https://doi.org/10.1136/bmjpo-2019-000592. PMID: 31909225; PMCID: PMC6936999
8. Arnts IJJ, Bullens LM, Groenewoud JMM, Liem KD. Comparison of complication rates between umbilical and peripherally inserted central venous catheters in newborns. J Obstet Gynecol Neonat Nurs. 2014;43(2):205–15.
9. Gordon A, Greenhalgh M, McGuire W. Early planned removal of umbilical venous catheters to prevent infection in newborn infants. Cochrane Database Syst Rev. 2017;10(10):CD012142. https://doi.org/10.1002/14651858.CD012142.pub2.
10. Lalitha R, Hicks M, Qureshi M, Kumaran K. Umbilical arterial catheter duration as risk factor for Bell's stage III necrotizing enterocolitis in preterm neonates. JPGN Rep. 2024;5:256–64. https://doi.org/10.1002/jpr3.12081.
11. Galdo F, Trappan A, Cossovel F, Rodriguez-Perez C, Ronfani L, Montaldo P, et al. Ultrasonographic measurements of the inferior vena cava diameter in newborns: is it a useful tool for choosing an umbilical venous catheter? Front Pediatr. 2023;11:1268622. https://doi.org/10.3389/fped.2023.1268622.
12. Barrington KJ. Umbilical artery catheters in the newborn: effects of position of the catheter tip. Cochrane Database Sys Rev 1999,2000;2:CD000505. doi:https://doi.org/10.1002/14651858.CD000505.
13. Seigel A, Evans N, Lutz T. Use of clinician-performed ultrasound in the assessment of safe umbilical venous catheter tip placement. J Paediatr Child Health. 2020;56(3):439–43. https://doi.org/10.1111/jpc.14658.

14. D'Andrea V, Prontera G, Pinna G, Cota F, Fattore S, Costa S, et al. Securement of umbilical venous catheter using cyanoacrylate glue: a randomized controlled trial. J Pediatr. 2023;260:113517. https://doi.org/10.1016/j.jpeds.2023.113517.

15. Perl JR, Crabtree-Beach T, Olyaei A, Hedges M, Jordan BK, Scottoline B. Reducing umbilical catheter migration rates by using a novel securement device. J Perinatol. 2024;44:1359. https://doi.org/10.1038/s41372-024-01943-1.

16. Anderson J, Leonard D, Braner DA, Lai S, Tegtmeyer K. Videos in clinical medicine. Umbilical vascular catheterization. N Engl J Med. 2008;359(15):e18. https://doi.org/10.1056/NEJMvcm0800666.

17. Julian S, Trivedi S, Vachharajani A. Video corner. Umbilical arterial catheterization. Neoreviews. 2016;17(12):e736–8. https://doi.org/10.1542/neo.17-12-e736.

18. Sobczak A, Dudzik A, Kruczek P, Kwinta P. Ultrasound monitoring of umbilical catheters in the neonatal intensive care unit—a prospective observational study. Front Pediatr. 2021;9:9. https://doi.org/10.3389/fped.2021.665214.

19. Franta J, Harabor A, Soraisham AS. Ultrasound assessment of umbilical venous catheter migration in preterm infants: a prospective study. Arch Dis Child Fetal Neonat Ed. 2017;102(3):F251–5. https://doi.org/10.1136/archdischild-2016-311202.

20. Rubortone SA, Costa S, Perri A, D'Andrea V, Vento G, Barone G. Real-time ultrasound for tip location of umbilical venous catheter in neonates: a pre/post intervention study. Ital J Pediatr. 2021;47(1):68. https://doi.org/10.1186/s13052-021-01014-7.

21. Tambasco CJ, Shabanova V, Peterec SM, BizzaroMJ. A novel and accurate method for estimating umbilical arterial and venous catheter insertion length. J Perinatol. 2021;41:1633–7. https://doi.org/10.1038/s41372-021-01121-7.

22. Sulemanji M, Vakili K, Zurakowski D, Tworetzky W, Fishman SJ, Kim HB. Umbilical venous catheter malposition is associated with necrotizing enterocolitis in premature infants. Neonatology. 2017;111(4):337–43.

23. Edison P, Arunachalam S, Baral V, Bharadwaj S. Varying clinical presentations of umbilical venous catheter extravasation: a case series. J Paediatr Child Health. 2021;57:1123–6. https://doi.org/10.1111/jpc.15137.

24. Gibson K, Sharp R, Ullman A, Morris S, Kleidon T, Esterman A. Adverse events associated with umbilical catheters: a systematic review and meta-analysis. J Perinatol. 2021;41:2505–12. https://doi.org/10.1038/s41372-021-01147-x.

25. Abdellatif M, Ahmed A, Alsenaidi K. Cardiac tamponade due to umbilical venous catheter in the newborn. BMJ Case Rep. 2012;2012:bcr-2012-6160. https://doi.org/10.1136/bcr-2012-6160.

26. Mense L, Rose S, Bruck A, Rüdiger M, Kaufmann M, Seipolt B. Peripheral arterial lines in extremely preterm neonates: a potential alternative to umbilical arterial catheters. Adv Neonat Care. 2022;22(4):357–61. https://doi.org/10.1097/ANC.0000000000000909.

27. Nobuo J, Tsunehiko S. Cannulation of the temporal artery in neonates and infants. Paediatr Anaesth. 2007;17(7):704–5. https://doi.org/10.1111/j.1460-9592.2006.02188.x.

28. Bruckner M, Schneider M, Reiterer F, Miledar LP, Baik-Schneditz N, Pichler G, et al. Peripheral arterial catheters in extremely preterm infants born at less than 28 weeks of gestation—a single-center experience. Eur J Pediatr. 2024;183:4345. https://doi.org/10.1007/s00431-024-05699-w.

29. Shah S, Kaul A, Mishra S, Pawale S. Clinical experience of use of percutaneous peripheral arterial cannulation in sick neonates in a developing country. BMC Pediatr. 2021;21(1):484. https://doi.org/10.1186/s12887-021-02943-2.

30. Schindler E, Kowald B, Suess H, Niehaus-Borquez B, Tausch B, Brecher A. Catheterization of the radial or brachial artery in neonates and infants. Paediatr Anaesth. 2005;15(8):677–82. https://doi.org/10.1111/j.1460-9592.2004.01522.x.

31. Dumond AA, da Cruz E, Almodovar MC, Friesen RH. Femoral artery catheterization in neonates and infants. Pediatr Crit Care Med. 2012;13(1):39–41. https://doi.org/10.1097/PCC.0b013e3182192c7b.

32. Fazan VP, Borges CT, Da Silva JH, Caetano AG, Filho OA. Superficial palmar arch: an arterial diameter study. J Anat. 2004;204(4):307–11. https://doi.org/10.1111/j.0021-8782.2004.00281.x.

33. Zarzecki MP, Popieluszko P, Zayachkowski A, Pękala PA, Henry BM, Tomaszewski KA. The surgical anatomy of the superficial and deep palmar arches: a meta-analysis. J Plast Reconstr Aesthet Surg. 2018;71(11):1577–92. https://doi.org/10.1016/j.bjps.2018.08.014.

34. Mavarez AC, Ripat C, Char S, Abuchaibe V, Galarza M, Halliday N, et al. Evaluation of distal radial artery cross-sectional internal diameter in neonates and infants by ultrasound and adequate selection of an intra-arterial catheter size. Paediatr Anaesth. 2021;31(12):1350–6. https://doi.org/10.1111/pan.14293.

35. Dasani R, Pai VV, Noh CY, Vallandingham-Lee S, Davis AS, Bhombal S. POCUS increases successful placement of peripheral arterial lines in neonates by less experienced providers. Eur J Pediatr. 2023;182(11):4977–82. https://doi.org/10.1007/s00431-023-05160-4.

36. Raphael CK, El Hage Chehade NA, Khabsa J, Akl EA, Aouad-Maroun M, Kaddoum R. Ultrasound-guided arterial cannulation in the paediatric population. Cochrane Database Syst Rev. 2023;3(3):CD011364. https://doi.org/10.1002/14651858.CD011364.pub3.

37. Wang Z, Guo H, Shi S, Xu Y, Ye M, Bai L, et al. Long-axis in-plane combined with short-axis out-of-plane technique in ultrasound-guided arterial catheterization in infants: a randomized controlled trial. J Clin Anesth. 2023;85:111038. https://doi.org/10.1016/j.jclinane.2022.111038.

38. Jang YE, Kim EH, Lee JH, Kim HS, Kim JT. Guidewire-assisted vs. direct radial arterial cannulation in neonates and infants: a randomised controlled trial. Eur J Anaesthesiol. 2019;36(10):738–44. https://doi.org/10.1097/EJA.0000000000001064.

39. Imbriaco G, Monesi A, Giugni A, Cilloni N. Radial artery cannulation in intensive care unit patients: does distance from wrist joint increase catheter durability and functionality? J Vasc Access. 2021;22(4):561–7. https://doi.org/10.1177/1129729820953020.

40. Spencer TR, Imbriaco G, Bardin-Spencer A, Mahoney KJ, Brescia F, Lamperti M, et al. Safe insertion of arterial catheters (SIA): an ultrasound-guided protocol to minimize complications for arterial cannulation. J Vasc Access. 2023;25:1403. https://doi.org/10.1177/11297298231178064.

41. Schults JA, Reynolds H, Rickard CM, Culwick MD, Mihala G, Alexandrou E, Ullman AJ. Dressings and securement devices to prevent complications for peripheral arterial catheters. Cochrane Database of Syst Rev. 2024;5:CD013023. https://doi.org/10.1002/14651858.CD013023.pub2.

42. Pearse I, Corley A, Bartnikowski N, Fraser JF. In vitro testing of cyanoacrylate tissue adhesives and sutures for extracorporeal membrane oxygenation cannula securement. Intensive Care Med Exp. 2021;9(1):5. https://doi.org/10.1186/s40635-020-00365-5.

43. Synnes AR, Reilly C, Robinson A. Limb length shortening associated with femoral arterial lines in the neonatal period. Paediatr Child Health. 2013;18(4):194–6. https://doi.org/10.1093/pch/18.4.194.

44. Turner L, Alexopolou V, Tawfik HTM, Silva M, Yoxall CW. Outcomes of femoral arterial catheterisation in neonates: a retrospective cohort study. Children (Basel). 2022;9(8):1259. https://doi.org/10.3390/children9081259.

45. Deindl P, Waldhör T, Unterasinger L, Berger A, Keck M. Arterial catheterisation in neonates can result in severe ischaemic complications but does not impair long-term extremity function. Acta Paediatr. 2018;107(2):240–8. https://doi.org/10.1111/apa.14100.

46. Kim J, Lee JW, Kim DY. Analysis of characteristics of peripheral arterial ischemia in premature babies and effects of nitroglycerin patch application. Child Health Nurs Res. 2020;26(4):434–44. https://doi.org/10.4094/chnr.2020.26.4.434.

47. Sushko K, Litalien C, Ferruccio L, Gilpin A, Mazer-Amirshahi M, Chan AK, et al. Topical nitroglycerin ointment as salvage therapy for peripheral tissue ischemia in newborns: a systematic review. CMAJ Open. 2021;9(1):E252–60. https://doi.org/10.9778/cmajo.20200129.

48. Mosalli R, Khayyat W, Al Qarni S, Al Matrafi A, El Baz M, Paes B. Topical nitroglycerin in newborns with ischemic injuries: a systematic review. Saudi Pharm J. 2021;29(7):764–74. https://doi.org/10.1016/j.jsps.2021.05.008.

49. Al Qurashi M, Al-Khotani A, Mohtisham F, AlRaddadi E, AlShaikh H, Hakami AY, Aga SS. Digital ischemia in an extreme preterm infant treated with nitroglycerin patch. Case Rep Pediatr. 2024;2024:2255756. https://doi.org/10.1155/2024/2255756.

50. De Carolis MP, Bersani I, Piersigilli F, Rubortone SA, Occhipinti F, Lacerenza S, et al. Peripheral nerve blockade and neonatal limb ischemia: our experience and literature review. Clin Appl Thromb Hemost. 2014;20(1):55–60. https://doi.org/10.1177/1076029612458968.

51. Piersigilli F, Bersani I, Giliberti P, Ronchetti MP, Mancinelli RL, Cavadenti I, et al. Neonatal limb ischemia: caudal blockade and NIRS monitoring. Eur J Pediatr. 2014;173(12):1599–601. https://doi.org/10.1007/s00431-013-2152-y.

52. DeBoer S, Russell T, Seaver M, Vardi A. Infant intraosseous infusion. Neonat Netw. 2008;27(1):25–32. https://doi.org/10.1891/0730-0832.27.1.25.

53. Schwindt E, Pfeiffer D, Gomes D, Brenner S, Schwindt JC, Hoffmann F, et al. Intraosseous access in neonates is feasible and safe—an analysis of a prospective nationwide surveillance study in Germany. Front Pediatr. 2022;10:952632. https://doi.org/10.3389/fped.2022.952632.

54. Mogale N, van Schoor AN, Bosman MC. A theoretical alternative intraosseous infusion site in severely hypovolemic children. Afr J Prim Health Care Fam Med. 2015;7(1):835. https://doi.org/10.4102/phcfm.v.7i1.835.

55. Mileder LP, Urlesberger B, Schwaberger B. Use of intraosseous vascular access during neonatal resuscitation at a tertiary center. Front Pediatr. 2020;8:571285. https://doi.org/10.3389/fped.2020.571285.

56. Scrivens A, Reynolds PR, Emery FE, Roberts CT, Polglase GR, Hooper SB, Roehr CC. Use of intraosseous needles in neonates: a systematic review. Neonatology. 2019;116(4):305–14. https://doi.org/10.1159/000502212.

57. Sengasai C, Pacharn P, Paes B, Kitsommart R. A prospective evaluation of tibial insertion sites for intraosseous needles to gain vascular access in Asian neonates. J Perinatol. 2024; https://doi.org/10.1038/s41372-024-02018-x.

58. Schwindt EM, Häcker T, Stockenhuber R, Patsch JM, Mehany SN, Berger A, et al. Finding the most suitable puncture site for intraosseous access in term and preterm neonates: an ultrasound-based anatomical pilot study. Eur J Pediatr. 2023;182(7):3083–91. https://doi.org/10.1007/s00431-023-04972-8.

59. Eifinger F, Scaal M, Wehrle L, Maushake S, Fuchs Z, Koerber F. Finding alternative sites for intraosseous infusions in newborns. Resuscitation. 2021;163:57–63. https://doi.org/10.1016/j.resuscitation.2021.04.004.

60. Oesterlie GE, Petersen KK, Knudsen L, Henriksen TB. Crural amputation of a newborn as a consequence of intraosseous needle insertion and calcium infusion. Pediatr Emerg Care. 2014;30(6):413–4. https://doi.org/10.1097/PEC.0000000000000150.

61. Ellemunter H, Simma B, Trawöger R, Maurer H. Intraosseous lines in preterm and full term neonates. Arch Dis Child Fetal Neonatal Ed. 1999;80(1):F74–5. https://doi.org/10.1136/fn.80.1.f74.

62. Elmitwalli I, Smith C, Tobias JD. Popliteal artery injury and loss of limb after intraosseous needle placement during resuscitation. Int J Clin Pediatri. 2023;12(1):22–7. https://www.theijcp.org/index.php/ijcp/article/view/511/432

63. Suominen PK, Nurmi E, Lauerma K. Intraosseous access in neonates and infants: risk of severe complications—a case report. Acta Anaesthesiol Scand. 2015;59(10):1389–93. https://doi.org/10.1111/aas.12602.

64. Molacek J, Houdek K, Opatny V, Fremuth J, Sasek L, Treskova I, et al. Serious complications of intraosseous access during infant resuscitation. Eu J Pediatr Surg Rep. 2018;6(1):e59–62. https://doi.org/10.1055/s-0038-1661407.

65. Raina R, Vijayaraghavan P, Kapur G, Sethi SK, Krishnappa V, Kumar D, et al. Hemodialysis in neonates and infants: a systematic review. Semin Dial. 2018;31(3):289–99. https://doi.org/10.1111/sdi.12657.

66. Mohamed TH, Morgan J, Mottes TA, Askenazi D, Jetton JG, Menon S. Kidney support for babies: building a comprehensive and integrated neonatal kidney support therapy program. Pediatr Nephrol. 2023;38(7):2043–55. https://doi.org/10.1007/s00467-022-05768-y.

67. Slagle C, Askenazi D, Starr M. Recent advances in kidney replacement therapy in infants: a review. Am J Kidney Dis. 2024;83(4):519–30. https://doi.org/10.1053/j.ajkd.2023.10.012.

68. Parolin M, Ceschia G, Vidal E. New perspectives in pediatric dialysis technologies: the case for neonates and infants with acute kidney injury. Pediatr Nephrol. 2024;39(1):115–23. https://doi.org/10.1007/s00467-023-05933-x.

69. Ree IMC, Besuden CFJ, Wintjens VEHJ, Verweij JEJT, Oepkes D, de Haas M, et al. Exchange transfusions in severe Rh-mediated alloimmune haemolytic disease of the foetus and newborn: a 20-year overview on the incidence, associated risks and outcome. Vox Sang. 2021;116(9):990–7. https://doi.org/10.1111/vox.13090.

70. Zwiers C, Slootweg YM, Koelewijn JM, Ligthart PC, van der Bom JG, van Kamp IL, et al. Disease severity in subsequent pregnancies with RhD immunization: a nationwide cohort. Vox Sang. 2024;119(8):859–66. https://doi.org/10.1111/vox.13651.

71. de Winter DP, Kaminski A, Tjoa ML, Oepkes D. Hemolytic disease of the fetus and newborn: systematic literature review of the antenatal landscape. BMC Pregnancy Childbirth. 2023;23(1):12. https://doi.org/10.1186/s12884-022-05329-z.

72. Alakhfash AA, Jelly A, Almesned A, Alqwaiee A, Almutairi M, Salah S, et al. Cardiac catheterisation in neonates and infants less than three months. J Saudi Heart Assoc. 2020;32(2):149–56. https://doi.org/10.37616/2212-5043.

73. Kang SL, Benson L. Recent advances in cardiac catheterization for congenital heart disease. F1000Res. 2018;7:370. https://doi.org/10.12688/f1000research.13021.1.

74. Fletcher K, Chapman R, Keene S. An overview of medical ECMO for neonates. Sem Perinatol. 2018;42(2):68–79. https://doi.org/10.1053/j.semperi.2017.12.002.

75. Van Ommen CH, Neunert CE, Chitlur MB. Neonatal ECMO. Front Med (Lausanne). 2018;5:289. https://doi.org/10.3389/fmed.2018.00289.

76. Rosario DC, Ambati S. Extracorporeal membrane oxygenation in children. [Updated 2023 Jul 10]. In: StatPearls [internet]. Treasure Island: StatPearls Publishing; 2024. https://www.ncbi.nlm.nih.gov/books/NBK572104/. Accessed 12 August 2024.

77. Wrisinger WC, Thompson SL. Basics of extracorporeal membrane oxygenation. Surg Clin North Am. 2022;102(1):23–35. https://doi.org/10.1016/j.suc.2021.09.001.

78. Robinson S, Peek G. The role of ECMO in neonatal and paediatric patients. Paediatri Child Health. 2019;29(5):218–23. https://doi.org/10.1016/j.paed.2019.02.004.

79. Etchill EW, Dante SA, Garcia AV. Extracorporeal membrane oxygenation in the pediatric population— who should go on, and who should not. Curr Opin Pediatr. 2020;32(3):416–23. https://doi.org/10.1097/MOP.0000000000000904.

80. Tonna JE, Boonstra PS, MacLaren G, Paden M, Brodie D, Anders M, et al. Extracorporeal life support organization registry international report 2022: 100,000 survivors. ASAIO J. 20241;70(2):131–43. doi:10.1097/MAT.0000000000002128.

81. Jensen AR, Davis C, Gray BW. Cannulation and decannulation techniques for neonatal ECMO. Semin Fetal Neonat Med. 2022;27(6):101404. https://doi.org/10.1016/j.siny.2022.101404.

82. Kipfmueller F, Bo B, Schmitt J, Sabir H, Schroeder L, Mueller A, et al. Percutaneous, ultrasound-guided single- and multisite cannulation for veno-venous extracorporeal membrane oxygenation in neonates. Pediatr Pulmonol. 2023;58(9):2574–82. https://doi.org/10.1002/ppul.26555.

83. Bianzina S, Singh Y, Iacobelli R, Amodeo A, Guner Y, Di Nardo M. Use of point-of-care ultrasound (POCUS) to monitor neonatal and pediatric extracorporeal life support. Eur J Pediatr. 2024;183(4):1509–24. https://doi.org/10.1007/s00431-023-05386-2.

84. Chernoguz A, Monteagudo J. Neonatal venoarterial and venovenous ECMO. Sem Pediatr Surg. 2023;32(4):151326. https://doi.org/10.1016/j.sempedsurg.2023.151326.

85. Pooboni SK, Gulla KM. Vascular access in ECMO. Indian J Thorac Cardiovasc Surg. 2021;37(Suppl 2):221–31. https://doi.org/10.1007/s12055-020-00999-w.
86. Church JT, Kim AC, Erickson KM, Rana A, Drongowski R, Hirschl RB, et al. Pushing the boundaries of ECLS: outcomes in <34 week EGA neonates. J Pediatr Surg. 2017;52(11):1810–5. https://doi.org/10.1016/j.jpedsurg.2017.03.054.
87. United Nations Convention on the Rights of the Child, (UNCRC). (November 20th 1989). https://www.unicef.org.uk. Accessed 12 August 2024.

Part IV

Neonatal Vascular Access in Context

Integrating Neonatal Vascular Access and Neuroprotective Care

8

Chapter Learning Objectives

Upon completing this chapter, readers will be able to:

- Critically reflect on the impact of vascular access procedures on infants and their families.
  - In relation to the developing neonatal brain, the physical and emotional impacts of associated complications, and infant and family experience.
- Evaluate strategies and interventions aimed at minimising potential neurodevelopmental risks associated with neonatal vascular access procedures.
- Critically reflect on their own and their unit's vascular access practices and ways that they might be improved on
  - In relation to the potential for improved patient outcomes from better team-working and integrating vascular access within neuroprotective and family integration strategies.
- Advocate for routinely applying neuroprotective measures and integrating parents into neonatal vascular access.

8.1   Introduction

The increasing sophistication of vascular access and infusion therapies has played a crucial role in improving infant survival rates [1]. These advancements have been driven by research, technical innovations, and practical knowledge from diverse fields of study and healthcare practice. Infants in neonatal intensive care units (NICUs) present with unique challenges when it comes to obtaining vascular access and administering infusion therapies. These include engineering and technical limitations but also patient factors such as their small size, skin immaturity, and susceptibility to infection [2]. This chapter brings together the themes from this book on neonatal vascular access and explores how developmentally supportive and

© The Author(s), under exclusive license to Springer Nature
Switzerland AG 2024
M. R. van Rens, K. Hugill, *Vascular Access in Neonatal Nursing Practice:*
A Neuroprotective Approach, https://doi.org/10.1007/978-3-031-81602-4_8

neuroprotective interventions can be applied to enhance infant well-being and improve outcomes for both infants and their families.

The aim of developmentally supportive and neuroprotective interventions is to create a calm and nurturing NICU environment that addresses the physical, social, psychological, and emotional needs of infants [3]. Environments guided by developmental models of care can foster parental presence and involvement, enhance healthcare provider well-being, and promote the best possible developmental outcomes for infants [4–7]. However, achieving these goals can be challenging. In daily clinical practice, healthcare providers often struggle to balance competing needs, priorities, and barriers to ensure that compassionate, equitable, and consistent care is provided [7–9]. By applying the knowledge and principles discussed throughout this book, healthcare professionals can work towards integrating neonatal vascular access with neuroprotective care, ultimately enhancing outcomes for both infants and their families.

8.2 The Origins of Parental Centeredness and Family Integration

The integration of parents into the care of their children in hospitals underwent dynamic changes in the mid-twentieth century, driven by theoretical developments and ethological and anthropological research. A key figure in this shift was psychotherapist John Bowlby, whose work for the World Health Organization (WHO) [10] was pivotal in challenging existing beliefs and introducing the essential concepts of *Attachment Theory*. In his book *Child Care and the Growth of Love* [11], Bowlby provided a psychological explanation of how human beings form enduring social bonds and how these bonds are affected by separation, loss, and grief [12]. This theory was later refined through empirical research by Bowlby, Mary Ainsworth, and others [13–16].

Parents naturally form powerful emotional connections with their infants. Establishing and maintaining these enduring social bonds requires reciprocity, proximity, and commitment [11, 12, 14]. However, the separation of parents and infants, particularly in hospital settings, can delay or interrupt this bonding process [14, 17, 18]. Attachment Theory, along with the simpler concept of *Bonding Theory* [17, 18], provides useful, albeit partial, explanations of how human relationships are formed and maintained. These concepts, though theoretically distinct have through the often synonymous use of the words 'bonding' and 'attachment,' become widely adopted terms in maternity and neonatal care.

In lay language, the terms 'attachment' and 'bonding' are often used interchangeably to describe parents' feelings of affection towards their infants. Although these terms simplify the theories, they offer a shared language that helps explain to parents why their involvement in caring for their infants is crucial. From a modern perspective, both theories have been critiqued for reflecting the dominant social norms of the time, particularly their exclusive focus on mother–infant relationships in traditional family structures. More recent iterations of these theories have become more inclusive. Despite these critiques, the application of attachment and bonding concepts in neonatal care continues to highlight the importance of delivering compassionate and humane care.

Research by James and Joyce Robertson, who used innovative methods to publicise their findings, confirmed the critical importance of parents' presence for their children. A notable example is their 1952 film 'A Two-Year-Old Goes to the Hospital' (available from www.concordmedia.org.uk) and the related publications [19]. The publicity generated by their work contributed to the paradigm shift in how child health services began to view parents [20]. However, the adoption of these changes in maternity and NICU settings often lagged behind those in other areas of child health. In neonatal care, influential publications [e.g., 21, 22] marked a transition to more inclusive ways of working across the globe.

The belief that parents are essential to high-quality care and optimal outcomes became foundational, and this principle continues to inform contemporary care models. Developmental care, family-centered care, and newer concepts like family-integrated care are now normative in shaping how neonatal services are organised and delivered (e.g., [4]).

8.2.1   Parents' Concerns

NICU patients are a heterogeneous group. Infants differ in terms of gestational age at birth, age since birth, birth weight and current weight, level of organ system maturation, developmental status, and pathology. All these factors directly affect vascular access practices. Despite the infant's condition or treatment requirements, there are always opportunities for parents to be involved in their care. International research and commentary over many years have consistently shown that for many parents, being present with their infant is an important first step in establishing emotional connectedness [5–7, 21–29]. This idea reflects how deeply ingrained the concepts of attachment and bonding are in everyday neonatal care [12, 14, 18, 22].

However, some parents find this involvement challenging for various reasons. These can include their own health status, other carer responsibilities, work or financial constraints, fear and their own emotional vulnerabilities.

Conversations with parents over the course of their NICU stay, informed by years of practice and research across the globe, reveal common concerns. Many parents enter the NICU in a state of shock and disbelief. As time passes, the ways in which parents express their worries can vary widely, influenced by factors such as culture, gender, perceived power relationships and their emotional state (Table 8.1).

Within individual families, parental priorities around the care of their infant can differ [30–35]. These differences can sometimes lead to disagreements amongst family members, and in rare cases, mediating such disputes can place nurses in challenging situations. In these instances, it is important for nurses to involve senior team members and establish a clear communication strategy from the outset. Importantly, parental disputes and differing priorities can often arise from different coping mechanisms in response of having an infant in the NICU.

Table 8.1 Worries frequently expressed by parents in NICUs

Will my baby die?
Can you make my baby better?
Don't let my baby feel pain
Is my baby getting the best treatment?
I don't know or understand what is happening?
Can I [touch, hold, feed, pray, bring grandparents, siblings, friends here, etc.]?
Will my baby grow to be healthy and normal?
When can we go home?

These disagreements may not always be directly related to the events in the NICU itself. Consequently, it is essential for nurses and other healthcare providers to remain aware of these dynamics when interacting with parents. Addressing concerns, responding to unasked questions at inappropriate times, or providing information prematurely can sometimes be poorly received. In such cases, it is always better to ask rather than make assumptions.

8.3   Doing Things to Help Integrate Vascular and Neuroprotective Care

Emotional reactions to stressful situations are deeply personal, subjective, and shaped by social and cultural contexts [36]. However, emotions are not static and change over time, influenced by factors such as age, environment, and social context [37]. Consequently, how individuals respond to stress can vary. In healthcare settings like NICUs, this variability necessitates individualised, tailored approaches to care. Each infant and family may require a unique response based on their emotional and situational needs.

8.3.1   Parents' Needs in Vascular Access

Current ideas in child healthcare confirm the view that parents want to be informed partners in providing care for their infant and in making decisions about that care [4, 5, 21, 22, 29, 31, 38, 39]. Parents often have specific individual needs related to vascular access that healthcare professionals must be aware of and address. These needs might include a history of adverse experiences with vascular access, needle phobia, or misunderstandings about procedures. Providing clear, accurate and understandable information about vascular access procedures, including their purpose, and potential risks, helps meet these needs. In addition to delivering information, offering emotional support to alleviate stress and fear, along with practical guidance, can empower parents to become appropriately involved in their infant's care. Addressing parents' needs requires a multifaceted approach. A comprehensive strategy may include interpersonal communication, the use of multimodal information delivery, skill-building and assessment, policy implementation, and role modelling by healthcare providers, as outlined in Text Box 8.1.

Text Box 8.1 Practice Point: A Multilevel Strategy for Infection Prevention
Parents should be made aware of the vulnerabilities to infection pertinent to
their infant and the measures taken by nurses and others to limit this risk.

- For example, verbally, in parent unit guides (hard copy and web based),
  posters.
- Doing this will help parents to become better acquainted with their infant.
- Parents and other family members (grandparents' siblings, etc.) should be
  taught how to wash their hands and perform hand hygiene correctly.
- Parents should be encouraged to remind healthcare providers to ensure that
  they have washed their hands/performed hand hygiene before touching
  their infant.
  - Parents might feel ill-equipped, uncertain, and unprepared to do this
    initially.
  - Nurses role modelling this behaviour and the respectful and receptive
    responses of those challenged will reassure parents and support their
    own endeavours in this regard.
- Consideration should be given as to how parent feedback on infection preven-
  tion can be incorporated into clinical audit cycles and quality improvement.
  - For example, modifying terms of reference to include parent represen-
    tation in groups and committees setting local clinical audit topics, or
    parents being routinely provided space to feedback on RCA investiga-
    tions concerning their infant.

8.3.1.1 Being Present

Facilitating and supporting parental presence and involvement provides a link
between parent outcomes and infant outcomes [4]. However, there is limited evidence regarding the optimal amount of parental presence or involvement. Figures
about the amount of time parents spend in the NICU vary internationally [40]. A
pan-European survey of 11 NICUs reported that median parental presence ranged
from 3.3 to 22.3 h per day. These figures were influenced by the availability of overnight accommodation for the parents but not by the distance from home to the unit
or the presence of other children in the family [40]. Notably, longer periods of
parental presence were associated with a statistically significant increase ($P < 0.001$)
in parent–infant skin-to-skin contact, ranging from 0.3 to 6.6 h per day [40].

Stress, both parental and infant, can significantly affect the vascular access process and the infant's subsequent neuroprotection. Increased parental stress levels can
influence decision-making, their presence on the NICU, communication with healthcare professionals, and their ability to provide care for their infant [32, 33, 41–45].
Addressing parental stress and providing appropriate education and support can foster a more positive and collaborative experience during vascular access procedures,
ultimately contributing to better long-term mental health outcomes [34, 42, 43].

Many interventions for parents focus upon reducing emotional stress, relationship building, and promoting physical and emotional closeness. Benzies et al. [31]
in a systematic review identified three common elements incorporated into successful parenting interventions. These were

- Using multiple component psychological support strategies
  - To help individuals manage their own stress and promote self-efficacy
- Providing education and coaching input for staff and parents
  - To create greater understanding and sensitivity towards other viewpoints and the needs of different people (e.g., staff and parents, parents with each other and different family members)
- Using therapeutic developmental interventions for infants to provide a pathway for parental engagement

8.3.1.2 Communicating

Parents who are overly suspicious of staff interfere with equipment, hover around the NICU (away from their infant), listening in to other people's conversations, or continually challenge staff can be perceived as problematic [46–48]. Difficult parent–staff interactions can also arise during discussions of medically complex illnesses, end-of-life care, or after a complaint or medical error. Staff judgments about families, particularly those with safeguarding issues, differing lifestyles, or self-identities that contrast with their own can lead to hostility and communication breakdowns [48, 49].

Effective communication is a foundational issue for the delivery of quality care. Despite its importance, poor communication remains one of the top concerns for patients and families [50]. Communication failures are frequently cited in root cause analyses of adverse healthcare events and complaints [51]. A report into complaints concerning doctors' communication identified four common failures:

1. Not providing timely information
2. Failing to share appropriate information with others
3. Not listening to patients
4. Not working in partnership with patients their family/carers

This review also identified 19 contributory factors, with the four most prominent being patient factors, staff workload, communication systems, and team factors [52]. Neonatal care is not immune to these communication challenges.

Effective communication with parents effectively is a core component of family-centered care [3, 21, 29, 31, 41, 45]. How nurses and other healthcare providers behave is critical to providing emotional, psychological, and informational support in a timely and effective manner. Fenwick et al. [53] highlighted the potential for using informal speech for parental support. However, casual conversations can be problematic in some situations. In emotionally charged environments, words and language can carry meaning beyond their immediate intent. Well-intentioned but poorly chosen remarks intended to provide comfort can reinforce parents 'wishful narratives' rather than addressing the reality of the situation [54]. This can be unhelpful, potentially affecting relationships and trust [54, 55].

Nurses play a core role in helping parents cope emotionally and navigate their NICU experience. Providing accurate, clear, information that is honest and strikes the right balance between professionalism and empathy can be helpful in individualising care, reinforcing personhood and humanising the behaviours of others (Text Box 8.2).

Text Box 8.2 Patient Views About Their Vascular Access

Patients' perspectives about the quality of care they receive around vascular access and infusion therapy are rarely sought or given prominence [56, 57].

- Infants in NICU are unable to express their thoughts about vascular access.
- Instead, nurses rely on proxy measures, or projection/transference of their own feelings and attitudes to understand their possible perspectives.

One hermeneutic phenomenological study explored the experiences of a group of adult participants (n = 15) receiving cancer care.

- Participants were asked to describe what it was like for them to be repeatedly cannulated.

Findings suggest that a paternalistic stance predominated, and a holistic approach to care was often missing causing the participants to feel vulnerable [56].

This insight is important for neonatal vascular access:

- It emphases the negative effects on patients lived experiences of solely focusing on the procedural task.
- It provides evidence for the need to take a more holistic approach that incorporates shared decision-making to vascular access.

Healthcare professionals should ensure that explanations provided to parents are tailored to their level of understanding and emotional readiness. When done effectively, this approach can alleviate anxiety, improve parental satisfaction, and empower parents to actively participate in decision-making. It also enables parents to advocate for their infant's comfort and safety, fostering a more collaborative and holistic approach to vascular access.

8.3.2   Infants' Needs in Vascular Access

It is impossible to know precisely what individual infants experience during vascular access procedures. However, it can be assumed that the absence of stress and pain, along with feeling safe and comforted, are key needs for infants.

8.3.2.1 Relieving Pain and Stress

Everyday stresses and exposure to noxious stimuli during the neonatal period can have profound effects on brain health and development [58–60]. In infants, stress responses during vascular access procedures can be triggered by factors such as pain, physical discomfort, and separation from familiar voices, touch, and odours. These stressors can lead to physiological changes, including increased heart rate, elevated blood pressure, and heightened cortisol levels, all of which can impact cerebral blood flow regulation. Minimising infant stress during vascular access is therefore crucial for maintaining neuroprotection [58].

Numerous neonatal pain assessment tools exist in the literature [61]. Proponents state that these tools can reduce the subjectivity of pain assessment and provide insight into an infant's response to pain relief. However, some tools are overly simplistic, unable to differentiate between stress and pain responses, or require long observation times and extensive training to ensure interrater reliability. This can lead to inconsistent or uncertain results. Despite these limitations, pain assessment tools play an important role in informing nurses about the presence of pain and the effectiveness of pain relief measures. Furthermore, they can serve as valuable tools to help parents understand their infant's behaviour, reinforcing the importance of pain prevention and alleviation as a critical clinical concern. One readily understandable way to consider the complex issues around the treatment of neonatal pain and embed pain prevention into everyday thinking is conveyed in the '*Ow Model*', a model based on combining the principles of empathy and patient rights (Text Box 8.3).

Text Box 8.3 Practice Point: The Ow Model
The central premise of this model is simple and relies on empathy and notions of patient rights.

If I think what I am about to experience might hurt me, cause me discomfort, or frighten me, then it will almost certainly be same for others.

If this is the case, I would want to:

- Avoid the pain
- Be comforted
- Be reassured
- And avoid the experience unless it was necessary for my well-being.

Surely, this is the minimum level of human empathy that we owe people* in our care.

*The word people is used purposefully to prompt consideration of obvious patient needs but also those of parents, colleagues, and others nearby who might be involved or witness our behaviours and actions.

Managing procedural pain in NICUs is widely considered challenging. However, there is a considerable body of evidence that underpins the efficacy of non-pharmacological measures. These interventions used alone or in combination with additional sensory inputs and environmental modifications can help infant self-regulation, reduce stress, decrease pain, and promote comfort [23, 24, 61–66]. Fostering parental involvement and support is vital for mitigating stress levels and ensuring a positive experience for both the neonate and parents [6, 29, 41, 67].

Kangaroo mother care (KMC, KC) and parent–infant, skin-to-skin contact are one of the key neuroprotective and developmentally supportive interventions supported by robust evidence for its effectiveness [23–26]. The benefits of skin-to-skin contact might be accumulative [41], although further research is required to confirm this. Organisational measures such as providing parents with overnight accommodation and domestic facilities can significantly increase the amount of time infants receive this intervention [40]. With some minor modifications to working practices, KMC can be integrated in many aspects of neonatal vascular access [26]. Doing this can provide an important means of providing comfort and an effective non-pharmacological measure for pain relief.

8.3.3   Organisational Needs in Vascular Access

8.3.3.1 Teamworking

An increasing body of empirical data from across different international healthcare settings supports the idea that specialist multi-professional team based vascular access approaches are superior to more generalist models in some important quality measures [68–71]. Neonatal-specific research into the benefits of peripheral and central vascular access teams confirms the benefits in connection with more consistent use of evidence-based practices, reduced incidence of phlebitis, lower bloodstream infection rates, higher first-attempt success rates, and overall fewer complications [72–74]. Despite these benefits, there remains a lack of consensus about the optimal composition of vascular access teams [70], and agreement on what are the most important outcomes to judge success [68].

8.3.3.2 Appling Health Technology

Smart infusion pumps have the potential to enhance patient safety, but only when used correctly. Errors occur at the interface of human factors and technology. These human factors include user knowledge, understanding, behaviour, fatigue, workload, and patient variability. Establishing robust operational protocols and guidelines and auditing compliance can be helpful in reducing error [75].

Information technology applications for smartphones are increasingly available to inform and guide clinical decisions. Examples of apps with vascular access content include: DavEXPERT (http://davexpert.gaveceIt.it), NeoMate (Neomate Ltd.), UmbiCalc (Yale New Haven Health), IFDC (Imperial College Healthcare NHS Trust), and Badger Link (Clevermed Ltd.). As this is a largely emergent and lightly regulated area of healthcare technology, nurses should exercise caution when choosing or using such applications, to date few have been formally evaluated.

Technologies like the ivWatch sensor system, though sophisticated, require minimal user training and only minor adjustments in working methods. Evidence from neonatal studies (e.g., [76–78]) convincingly demonstrates the device's potential to provide earlier infiltration notifications and reduce the severity of these events. Point-of-care ultrasound has established itself as a novel but increasingly important tool in neonatology. It is used in an increasing array of clinical applications [79], indeed by some measures it has displaced some of the older tools of medicine.

Ultrasound monitoring in intensive care units has become the stethoscope of the 21st century [80].

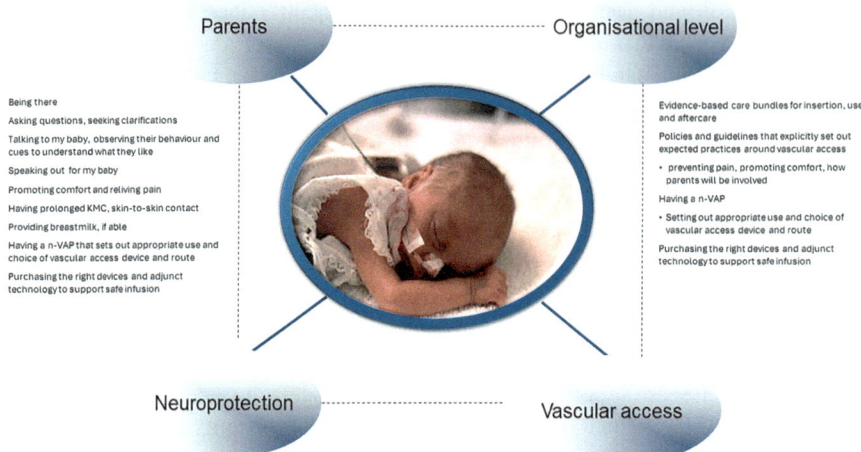

Fig. 8.1 Things that help. (The central image shows one of the author's own children born at 32 weeks gestation over 35 years ago. The MARSI from nasogastric tube taping is long resolved, but she still has faintly visible scars (more noticeable on tanning) from vascular access on her wrists and ankles.)

During vascular access, real-time ultrasound is becoming an essential tool for systematic and objective pre-procedural vascular assessment, site selection, insertion, catheter navigation and tip locating, and catheter tip surveillance. This shift in practice necessitates a programme of targeted education and training for nurses and other healthcare providers involved in obtaining vascular access [81–83].

Locally delivered training using multimodal pedagogical strategies in the use of real-time ultrasound can significantly impact both practice and patient care [82, 84]. For example, Rubortone et al. [84] report that after such training, the use of bedside ultrasound increased and UVC tips were more frequently correctly placed (75% vs. 30.7%, $p = 0.0023$). This improvement offers several patient benefits, including reduced exposure to X-rays, fewer failed insertions, less handling, and less catheter manipulation.

Figure 8.1 summarises organisational and parent level strategies and interventions that can help to better integrate neuroprotection and vascular access.

8.3.4   Looking to the Future

8.3.4.1 Artificial Intelligence in Healthcare

Artificial intelligence (AI) in healthcare has the potential to enhance clinical effectiveness, reduce errors, and improve care and treatment options [85]. It is important to recognise that AI is not a singular entity; instead, it is categorised based on functionality, system type, and levels of intelligence [86]. Two main categories of AI are defined based on intelligence levels:

- Narrow intelligence: These systems are designed to perform specific tasks. All current AI systems fall under this category.
- General intelligence: These systems can perform multiple tasks simultaneously and make independent decisions. In its most advanced form, such a system would be able to think like a human and could even possess self-awareness.

Alternatively, AI systems can be classified by system type:

- Reactive systems: These respond to external stimuli to prompt specific actions. They do not form memories and are incapable of learning.
- Limited memory systems: The most common type used in commerce and research, these systems possess memory and can build on available data to make future predictions and guide their actions.

The next two categories are mostly theoretical at this point:

- Theory of mind systems: These could potentially identify and respond to human emotions.
- Self-aware systems: In their most advanced form, these systems would not only recognise emotions but also experience their own emotions, desires, and goals.

In healthcare, a range of narrow limited-memory AI systems are currently being investigated or implemented. For example, they are used in patient monitoring systems, such as predictive algorithms for morbidity using real-time data (e.g., CTG interpretation and ECG signal analysis to predict infection risks) [85–87].

Role-based expert systems employing machine learning are also being developed to assist with diagnostics (especially in medical image interpretation), as well as healthcare logistics management and billing [87]. Although future developments are still speculative, they could include innovations such as robot-assisted surgery and the analysis of large datasets in fields like epidemiology or drug research [86]. In vascular access training, advancements in simulation using augmented reality with realistic, real-time feedback would be a valuable addition to support training [88].

8.3.4.2 Artificial Womb Technology

Recently, long-standing ideas about how to provide an extra uterine life support systems (ECLS) for those born at or below the current margins of viability have progressed. In part this has been due to developments in physiological management, vascular access, and the miniaturisation of existing extracorporeal tissue oxygenation technologies. Artificial womb technology (AWT) seeks to replicate the natural uterine environment amniotic sac. This technology is distinct from parallel development of the artificial placenta (AP) [89–91].

This rapid development has raised the prospect of considerable ethical and legal challenges concerning personhood and abortion rights [92, 93]. Romanis [93] contends that individuals experiencing AWT are legally and ethically neither foetus nor newborn infant. The term 'gestateling' is proposed to frame ethical discussions.

Central to this debate is, is AWT an extension of current life-preserving approaches or something new? Answering this question will necessitate a paradigm shift in the way treatment of infants born at the very margins of current viability is managed. Though this is likely some way off, there is a need to examine the scientific differences between AP and AWT and address the current lack of guidelines for study design, participant enrolment and eligibility, and research ethics [92]. If this technology develops into an acceptable and viable treatment option in the future, safe and effective vascular access will be essential.

8.4 Final Thoughts

The incidence of preterm birth has largely remained static over the past decade [94]. However, the demographic profile of infants admitted to NICUs in many countries is changing. In part, this reflects the potential for survival from improvements in treatment. However, this development is bringing about newer clinical, technical, and engineering challenges for vascular access as smaller infants at younger gestational ages survive.

Ideas and practices around developmental and neuroprotective care have global relevance and are bound in cultural notions and ideas about the nature and desirability of parental involvement. Early ideas about supportive interventions were based on theoretical developments and the principles of beneficence. When collectively integrated into everyday practice, neuroprotective and developmentally supportive interventions can reduce pain and stress, promote infant self-regulation, support parental presence, participation, the forming of emotional attachments, and improve important clinical, psychological, and quality of life outcome measures [3–7, 21–27, 95–99].

8.4.1 Questions for Research

The skilful insertion, use, and care of vascular access devices impacts immediate and longer term outcomes for infants but also lays the foundations for healthier futures for them and their families [2]. However, there remains many uncertainties in practice which future research could seek to answer. Nursing research into neonatal vascular access, developmentally supportive and neuroprotective interventions is an expanding field of study, with its own distinctive agendas. Yet, there has been limited exploration of the potential synergies between the two areas. This gap in research is to the detriment of infants in NICUs. Elevating the profile of vascular access and its connections to neuroprotection and improved outcomes could help bridge this gap and improve care.

Nurses work with real people in real-world settings, so nursing research must take an eclectic and holistic approach to generating new knowledge and applying it to evidence-based practice. This approach is both a strength and a challenge.

Determining optimal neonatal vascular practice is often hindered by insufficient or inconclusive research evidence, making it challenging to offer clear recommendations for practice. Throughout the preparation of this book, several questions have arisen that warrant further investigation and empirical study. Many of these questions could guide future research agendas, with Table 8.2 offering examples to stimulate further thought.

Table 8.2 Sample future research questions

Parental involvement and communication
How best to involve parents in vascular access procedures?
What role can digital tools (e.g., telemedicine, AI-assisted communication platforms) play in enhancing parental involvement and decision-making?

Pain management and procedural optimisation
What are the optimal combinations of non-pharmacological and pharmacological interventions for procedural pain associated with vascular access?
How can AI algorithms be used to develop personalised pain management plans?

Vascular access techniques and safety
What are the optimal vascular access routes, devices, insertion techniques, securement, and exit site protection strategies for specific patient and therapy circumstances?
How can AR (augmented reality) be used to enhance vein visualisation and catheter pathways?
Can point-of-care ultrasound technology combined with AI algorithms improve the precision of catheter placement and reduce procedural errors?
How best to reduce the incidence of complications, their number, nature, and severity?
Can continuous monitoring systems combined with AI-based predictive models prevent vascular access complications?

Skin protection and adhesive safety
Which tissue adhesive formulations are safe to use on neonatal skin?

How can smart materials and integrated sensors help monitor skin integrity in neonates?
Modifiable factors and team efficiency
Which potentially modifiable factors contribute most to improved vascular access?
What outcomes are the most important for vascular access teams to focus upon?
What is the ideal membership of vascular access teams?
Can AI-driven scheduling and team management tools optimise the deployment of vascular access teams?

Neonatal vascular access management plan (n-VAMP)
What are the essential components of an n-VAMP?
How can AI-based decision support systems assist in modifying n-VAMPs in real-time?

Healing environment and neuroprotective measures
What constitutes a 'healing environment'?
How can virtual reality (VR) and augmented reality (AR) technologies be used to create calming, neuroprotective environments for neonates during vascular access?

Training and simulation
How can augmented reality (AR) be integrated into neonatal vascular access training?
Can AI and machine learning models be utilised to simulate neonatal vascular access scenarios and provide real-time feedback for healthcare provider training?

Post-procedural monitoring
How can wearable technologies and biosensors improve post-procedural monitoring in neonates?
Can smart sensors provide continuous, real-time data on catheter function and potential complications?

Whilst this list of sample question is not exhaustive, it serves to demonstrate the scope of opportunities available.

8.4.2 Bringing It all Together and Defragmenting Care

Chapter 2 drew attention to the risks for infants, their families, nurses, and organisations from isolating vascular access from wider care concerns leading to a fragmentation in care (Fig. 2.3, Chap. 2). Successfully integrating vascular access and neuroprotective measures involves the assimilation of diverse fields of knowledge and skills and can help to defragment care (Fig. 8.2) and achieve potentially better outcomes for infants and their families. This book provides valuable insights into this complex topic, raising awareness for the need for a considered, proactive and informed approach that underpins ethical decision-making and the defragmentation of care (Text Box 8.4).

Text Box 8.4 Practice Point: Ensuring Safe Vascular Access, Essential Questions
Do I need to do this needlestick or venipuncture?

- Consider the alternatives you have considered and ruled out.

What can I do to make this procedure less painful and more successful?

- Consider infant sleep wake cycle, behavioural cues, clinical urgency.

What comfort promoting and pain reliving interventions am I going to use?

- Consider, what can the infant's parents do to contribute to minimising the pain and stress of this procedure.

How will I know if the interventions I am going to use are effective?

- Consider, possible use of formal pain scoring tools, infant behavioural responses, intuitive knowledge.

Am I familiar with using the device and insertion technique?
Do I know when to stop?

- Consider, have you demonstrated competence to undertake this task? if so,

Do I need assistance?

- Yes always

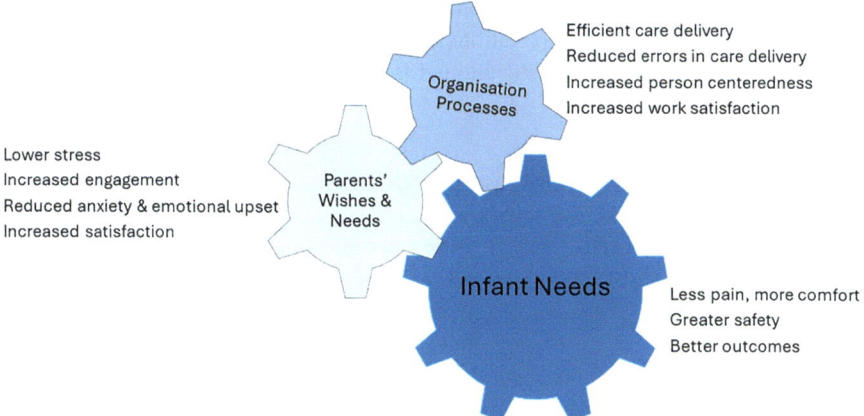

Fig. 8.2 Defragmenting care—meeting infant needs by synchronising care with parent wishes and organisation processes

Key Points

Parents' perspectives on neonatal vascular access are influenced by their emotional attachments and previous life experience around vascular access.

Parents have specific needs related to vascular access, including access to clear and understandable information, emotional support, and involvement in decision-making.

Effective communication and information sharing are essential for ensuring safe vascular access.

Parents prioritise minimising pain and discomfort for their child during vascular access procedures.

Involving parents in the vascular access process through family-integrated care enhances parental satisfaction, promotes shared decision-making, and strengthens the parent–infant attachments.

Parental involvement fosters a collaborative approach to care, where parents can contribute their unique insights and advocate for their child's well-being.

Healthcare professionals should prioritise safety, efficacy, and individualised care when performing vascular access procedures.

Point-of-care ultrasound for pre-procedural assessment, device insertion, catheter navigation, and tip location and surveillance is becoming the new 'gold standard' in vascular access practice.

Non-pharmacological comfort measures can be effective at reducing stress, relieving pain, and promoting postprocedure recovery.

There are numerous uncertainties about best practices which future research could seek to answer.

Integrating neuroprotective and developmentally supportive measures with vascular access can help to defragment care delivery and experience.

Reflective Activity: A Former Patient's Perspectives on Care At the beginning of this book, we set out our motivations for embarking on this endeavour. This was not the whole story. The following anonymised and abridged account is part of one former NICU patient's story.

Occasionally, former patients visit the NICU. One day, a young adult called Stella accompanied by her social worker had arranged to visit. It was delegated to me to meet with her and answer her questions.

Many years previously Stella had spent time on this unit. Stella wanted to know more about her early life as she was about to leave foster care and lacked this information. During conversation, it emerged that she had been born at 27 weeks weighing around 1.2 kg; she was in fact a remarkable survivor from the pre-surfactant era. However, all was not good. Stella showed me her arms, she had numerous scars (with more, she said in her hair, ankles, and the side of her chest).

I explained the possible causes. Looking at her arms, it seemed likely they were associated with vascular access, whilst the location of those on her thorax was possibly related to chest drains.

Stella seemed happy with my explanations about her scarring, I asked her why? She explained that at school, she had being labelled for 'self-harming' and had experienced stigma and discrimination because of this. A situation made worse for her by not knowing why she had these scars and been unable to refute this false allegation. However, now she knew why she had these 'survivor's marks' a weight had been lifted from her worries.

Throughout this book, we have used case histories based on real-life events to stimulate thought and reflection and provide an opportunity for readers to relate them to their own practice experiences. This final reflective case concerns a chance encounter which had a profound effect on the author's thinking about the many ways we unknowingly influence the futures of infants and their families in our care.

Over to You, Constructing Your Own Case
Thinking about your vascular access related experiences, identify an occasion where your experience was especially memorable (either positive or negative).

1. What factors made this event especially memorable to you?
2. How would you define a good or bad vascular access experience?
   (a) Consider who was it bad or good for and why.
       (i) Who, you, the infant or their parents.
       (ii) Why, ease or success of insertion or failure, confidence building or damaging, the amount of pain experienced, successful therapy delivery, life-saving effects, relaying bad news, complications and their aftereffects, etc.

3. Considering your own experiences and the recollections in the above case what arrangements are in place in your place of work to support safe vascular access, do these work and how can they be improved upon?

References

1. Christie DA, Tansey EM, editors. Welcome witness to twentieth century medicine: origins of neonatal intensive care in the UK (9). London: Welcome Trust Centre at University College; 2001. https://wellcomecollection.org/works/znbxa5qs. Accessed 12 August 2024
2. van Rens MFPT, Hugill K, Mahmah MA, Bayoumi M, Francia ALV, Garcia KLP, et al. Evaluation of unmodifiable and potentially modifiable factors affecting peripheral intravenous device-related complications in neonates: a retrospective observational study. BMJ Open. 2021;11(9):e047788. https://doi.org/10.1136/bmjopen-2020-047788.
3. Byers JF. Components of developmental care and the evidence for their use in the NICU. Am J Mat Child Nurs. 2003;28(3):174–80. https://doi.org/10.1097/00005721-200305000-00007.
4. British Association of Perinatal Medicine (BAPM). Family integrated care a framework for practice. London: BAPM; 2021. https://www.bapm.org/resources/ficare-framework-for-practice. Accessed 12 August 2024
5. Thomson G, Hall-Moran V, Axelin A, Dykes F, Flacking R. Integrating a sense of coherence into the neonatal environment. BMC Pediatr. 2013;13(84) https://doi.org/10.1186/1471-2431-13-84.
6. European Foundation for the Care of newborn infants, (EFCNI). Infant and family-centered developmental care. European standards of care for newborn health. Munich: EFCNI: 2018.. https://newborn-health-standards.org/downloads/. Accessed 12 August 2024.
7. Westrup B, Stjernqvist K, Kleberg A, Hellström-Westas L, Lagercrantz H. Neonatal individualized care in practice: a Swedish experience. Semin Neonatol. 2002;7(6):447–57. https://doi.org/10.1053/siny.2002.0150.
8. van der Pal SM, Maguire CM, Cessie SL, Veen S, Wit JM, Walther FJ, et al. Staff opinions regarding the newborn individualized developmental care and assessment program (NIDCAP). Early Hum Dev. 2007;83(7):425–32. https://doi.org/10.1016/j.earlhumdev.2007.03.007.
9. Mosqueda R, Castilla Y, Perapoch J, de la Cruz J, López-Maestro M, Pallás C. Staff perceptions on newborn individualized developmental care and assessment program (NIDCAP) during its implementation in two Spanish neonatal units. Early Hum Dev. 2013;89(1):27–33. https://doi.org/10.1016/j.earlhumdev.2012.07.013.
10. Bowlby J. Maternal care and maternal mental health. Geneva: World Health Organisation, (WHO); 1951.
11. Bowlby J. Child care and the growth of love. 2nd ed. Harmondsworth: Penguin; 1965.
12. Bowlby J. The making and breaking of affectional bonds. London: Routledge Classics; 1979, 2005.
13. Bowlby J. A secure base: clinical applications of attachment theory. London: Routledge Classics; 1988,2005.
14. Ainsworth MS. Infant–mother attachment. Am Psychol. 1979;34(10):932–7.
15. Robertson J. Young children in hospital. 2nd ed. London: Tavistock Press; 1970.
16. Robertson J, Robertson J. Separation and the very young. London: Free Association Books; 1989.
17. Klaus MH, Kennell JH. Maternal-infant bonding. St Louis: CV Mosby; 1976.
18. Klaus MH, Kennell JH. Parent infant bonding. 2nd ed. St Louis: CV Mosby; 1982.
19. Robertson JP, Robertson JP. A two year old goes to the hospital, film. London: Concord Video and Film Council; 1953. www.concordmedia.org.uk. Accessed 12 August 2024

20. Lindsay B. 'A 2-year-old goes to hospital': a 50th anniversary reappraisal of the impact of James Robertson's film. J Child Health Care. 2003;7(1):17–26. https://doi.org/10.117 7/1367493503007001672.
21. Harrison H. The principles for family-centered neonatal care. Pediatr. 1993;92(5):643–50.
22. Als H, Gilkerson L. The role of relationship-based developmentally supportive newborn intensive care in strengthening outcome of preterm infants. Sem Perinatol. 1997;21(3):178–89.
23. Zengin H, Suzan OK, Hur G, Kolukisa T, Eroglu A, Cinar N. The effects of kangaroo mother care on physiological parameters of premature neonates in neonatal intensive care unit: a systematic review. J Pediatr Nurs. 2023;71:E18–27. https://doi.org/10.1016/j.pedn.2023.04.010.
24. Johnston C, Campbell-Yeo M, Disher T, Benoit B, Fernandes A, Streiner D, et al. Skin-to-skin care for procedural pain in neonates. Cochrane Database Syst Rev. 2017;2(2):CD008435. https://doi.org/10.1002/14651858.CD008435.pub3.
25. Charpak N, Tessier R, Ruiz JG, Hernandez JT, Uriza F, Villegas J, et al. Twenty-year follow-up of kangaroo mother care versus traditional care. Pediatr. 2017;139(1):e20162063. https://doi.org/10.1542/peds.2016-2063.
26. Sipkema P, Van Rens M, Hugill K. Maintaining parent-infant skin-to-skin contact during peripheral intravenous catheter insertion in a Dutch neonatal unit. J Neonat Nurs. 2024;30(4):393–7. https://doi.org/10.1016/j.jnn.2024.01.004.
27. Kim J. A concept analysis on the use of Yakson in the NICU. J Obstet Gynecol Neonat Nurs. 2016;45:836–41. https://doi.org/10.1016/j.jogn.2016.07.009.
28. Thomas LM. The changing role of parents in neonatal care: a historical review. Neonat Network. 2008;27(2):91–100.
29. Dunst CJ, Trivette CM, Deal AG. Enabling and empowering families: principles and guidelines for practice. Cambridge: Brookline; 1998.
30. Hugill K, Harvey M. Fatherhood in midwifery and neonatal practice. London: Quay; 2012.
31. Benzies KM, Magill-Evans JE, Hayden KA, Ballantyne M. Key components of early intervention programs for preterm infants and their parents: a systematic review and meta-analysis. BMC Pregnancy Childbirth. 2013;13(S1):S10. http://www.biomedcentral.com/1471-2393/13/S1/S10
32. Hagen IH, Iversen VC, Svindseth MF. Differences and similarities between mothers and fathers of premature children: a qualitative study of parents' coping experiences in a neonatal intensive care unit. BMC Pediatr. 2016;16:92. https://doi.org/10.1186/s12887-016-0631-9.
33. Ionio C, Colombo C, Brazzoduro V, Mascheroni E, Confalonieri E, Castoldi F, et al. Mothers and fathers in NICU: the impact of preterm birth on parental distress. Eur J Psychol. 2016;12(4):604–21. https://doi.org/10.5964/ejop.v12i4.1093.
34. Lakshmanan A, Agni M, Lieu T, Fleegler E, Kipke M, Friedlich PS, et al. The impact of preterm birth <37 weeks on parents and families: a cross-sectional study in the 2 years after discharge from the neonatal intensive care unit. Health Qual of Life Outcomes. 2017;15(1):38. https://doi.org/10.1186/s12955-017-0602-3.
35. Pace Parascandalo R, Hugill K. Supporting early parenting following preterm birth. In: Borg-Xuereb R, Jones J, editors. Perspectives in midwifery and parenthood. London: Springer; 2023. p. 83–94.
36. Hochschild AR. Emotion work, feeling rules, and social structure Am J Sciol. 1979;85(3):551–75.
37. Bolton SC. Emotion management in the workplace. Basingstoke: Palgrave; 2005.
38. Bliss. Bliss neonatal services for the future: a manifesto. (Nov. 2023). https://www.bliss.org.uk/research-campaigns/influencing-policy-and-working-in-parliament/future-neonatal-services. Accessed 12 August 2024.
39. iSupport Team. Editorial: getting it right first time and every time; re-thinking children's rights when they have a clinical procedure. J Pediatr Nurs. 2021;2021(61):A10–2. https://doi.org/10.1016/j.pedn.2021.11.017.
40. Raiskila S, Axelin A, Toome L, Caballero S, Tandberg BS, Montirosso R, et al. Parents' presence and parent-infant closeness in 11 neonatal intensive care units in six European countries vary between and within the countries. Acta Paediatr. 2017;106(6):878–88. https://doi.org/10.1111/apa.13798.

41. Horner S. Impact of parental presence and engagement on stress in NICU infants. Adv Neonat Care. 2024;24(2):132–40. https://doi.org/10.1097/ANC.0000000000001146.
42. Schecter R, Pham T, Hua A, Spinazzola R, Sonnenklar J, Li D, et al. Prevalence and longevity of PTSD symptoms among parents of NICU infants analyzed across gestational age categories. Clin Pediatr (Phila). 2020;59(2):163–9. https://doi.org/10.1177/0009922819892046.
43. McKeown L, Burke K, Cobham VE, Kimball H, Foxcroft K, Callaway L. The prevalence of PTSD of mothers and fathers of high-risk infants admitted to NICU: a systematic review. Clin Child Fam Psychol Rev. 2023;26(1):33–49. https://doi.org/10.1007/s10567-022-00421-4.
44. Voulgaridou A, Paliouras D, Deftereos S, Skarentzos K, Tsergoula E, Miltsakaki I, et al. Hospitalization in neonatal intensive care unit: parental anxiety and satisfaction. Pan Afr Med J. 2023;44:55. https://doi.org/10.11604/pamj.2023.44.55.34344.
45. Gallagher K, Shaw C, Aladangady N, Marlow N. Parental experience of interaction with healthcare professionals during their infant's stay in the neonatal intensive care unit. Arch Dis Child Fetal Neonat Ed. 2018;103(4):F343–8. https://doi.org/10.1136/archdischild-2016-312278.
46. Friedman J, Hatters Friedman S, Collin M, Martin RJ. Staff perceptions of challenging parent–staff interactions and beneficial strategies in the neonatal intensive care unit. Acta Paediatr. 2017;107(1):33–9. https://doi.org/10.1111/apa.14025.
47. Toren O, Nirel N, Tsur Y, Lipschuetz M, Toker A. Examining professional boundaries between nurses and physicians in neonatal intensive care units. Israel J Health Policy Res. 2014;3:43. http://www.ijhpr.org/content/3/1/43.
48. Hugill K. Father-staff relationships in a neonatal unit: being judged and judging. Infant. 2014;10(4):128–31.
49. Swedberg Yinger O, Jones A, Fallin-Bennett K, Gibbs C, Farr RH. Family-centered care for LGBTQ+ parents of infants in the neonatal intensive care unit: an integrative review. Children (Basel). 2024;11:615. https://doi.org/10.3390/children11060615.
50. O'Hara JK, Reynolds C, Moore S, Armitage G, Sheard L, March C, et al. What can patients tell us about the quality and safety of hospital care? Findings from a UK multicentre survey study. BMJ Qual Saf. 2018;27(9):673–82. https://doi.org/10.1136/bmjqs-2017-006974.
51. Dayton E, Henriksen K. Communication failure: basic components, contributing factors, and the call for structure. Joint Commission J Qual Patient Saf. 2005;33(1):34–47. https://doi.org/10.1016/S1553-7250(07)33005-5.
52. General Medical Council, (GMC). Communication complaint types and contributory factors. London: GMC; 2018. https://www.gmc-uk.org/-/media/documents/communication-complaint-types-and-contributory-factors-report_pdf-80571206.pdf. Accessed 12 August 2024.
53. Fenwick J, Barclay L, Schmied V. 'Chatting': an important clinical tool in facilitating mothering in neonatal nurseries. J Adv Nurs. 2001;33(5):583–93.
54. Magliyah AF, Razzak MI. The parents' perception of nursing support in their neonatal intensive care unit (NICU) experience. Int J Adv Computer Sci Applic. 2015;6(2):153–8. https://doi.org/10.14569/IJACSA.2015.060222.
55. Bry A, Wigert H. Psychosocial support for parents of extremely preterm infants in neonatal intensive care: a qualitative interview study. BMC Psychol. 2019;7:76. https://doi.org/10.1186/s40359-019-0354-4.
56. Robinson-Reilly M, Paliadelis P, Cruickshank M. Venous access: the patient experience. Support Care Cancer. 2016;24(3):1181–7. https://doi.org/10.1007/s00520-015-2900-9.
57. Wheeler C, Furniss D, Galal-Edeen GH, Blandford A, Franklin BD. Patients' perspectives on the quality and safety of intravenous infusions: a qualitative study. J Patient Exp. 2020;7(3):380–5. https://doi.org/10.1177/2374373519843921.
58. van Dokkum NH, de Kroon MLA, Reijneveld SA, Bos AF. Neonatal stress, health, and development in preterms: a systematic review. Pediatr. 2021;148(4):e2021050414. https://doi.org/10.1542/peds.2021-050414.
59. Zhao T, Griffith T, Zhang Y, Li H, Hussain N, Lester B, et al. Early-life factors associated with neurobehavioral outcomes in preterm infants during NICU hospitalization. Pediatr Res 2022;92:1695–704. https://doi.org/10.1038/s41390-022-02021-y.

60. Selvanathan T, Miller SP. Brain health in preterm infants: importance of early-life pain and analgesia exposure. Pediatr Res. 2024;96:1397. https://doi.org/10.1038/s41390-024-03245-w.
61. Campbell-Yeo M, Eriksson M, Benoit B. Assessment and management of pain in preterm infants: a practice update. Children (Basel). 2022;9(2):244. https://doi.org/10.3390/children9020244.
62. Badiee Z, Asghari M, Mohammadizadeh M. The calming effect of maternal breast milk odor on premature infants. Pediatr Neonat. 2013;54:322–5. https://doi.org/10.1016/j.pedneo.2013.04.004.
63. Fitri SYR, Wardhani V, Rakhmawati W, Pahria T, Hendrawati S. Culturally based practice in neonatal procedural pain management: a mini review. Front Pediatr. 2020;8:540. https://doi.org/10.3389/fped.2020.00540.
64. Hoarau K, Payet ML, Zamidio L, Bonsante F, Iacobelli S. 'Holding–cuddling' and sucrose for pain relief during venepuncture in newborn infants: a randomized, controlled trial (CÂSA). Front Pediatr. 2021;8:607900. https://doi.org/10.3389/fped.2020.607900.
65. Shiff I, Bucsea O, Pillai RR. Psychosocial and neurobiological vulnerabilities of the hospitalized preterm infant and relevant non-pharmacological pain mitigation strategies. Front Pediatr. 2021;9:568755. https://doi.org/10.3389/fped.2021.568755.
66. Carozza S, Leong V. The role of affectionate caregiver touch in early neurodevelopment and parent–infant interactional synchrony. Front Neurosci. 2021;14:613378. https://doi.org/10.3389/fnins.2020.613378.
67. Ullsten A, Campbell-Yeo M, Eriksson M. Parent-led neonatal pain management-a narrative review and update of research and practices. Front Pain Res (Lausanne). 2024;5:1375868. https://doi.org/10.3389/fpain.2024.1375868.
68. Marsh N, Larsen E, Webster J, Cooke M, Rickard CM. The benefit of a vascular access specialist placing a peripheral intravenous catheter: a narrative review of the literature. Vasc Access. 2020;6(1):10–5. https://doi.org/10.33235/va.6.1.10-15.
69. Ríos LR, Català EC, Calsapeu PA, Mas AC, Martínez AI, Ruiz NI, et al. Implementation of a vascular access specialist team in a tertiary hospital: a cost-benefit analysis. Cost Eff Resour Alloc. 2023;21(1):67. https://doi.org/10.1186/s12962-023-00464-6.
70. Carr PJ, Higgins NS, Cooke ML, Mihala G, Rickard CM. Vascular access specialist teams for device insertion and prevention of failure. Cochrane Database Syst Rev. 2018;3(3) CD011429 https://doi.org/10.1002/14651858.CD011429.pub2.
71. Nickel B, Gorski L, Kleidon T, Kyes A, DeVries M, Keogh S, et al. Infusion therapy standards of practice. 9th ed. J Inf Nurs 2024;47(1S): S1–285. doi:https://doi.org/10.1097/NAN.0000000000000532.
72. Bayoumi MAA, Van Rens MFP, Chandra P, Francia ALV, D'Souza S, George M, et al. Effect of implementing an epicutaneo-caval catheter team in neonatal intensive care unit. J Vasc Access. 2020;22(2):243–53. https://doi.org/10.1177/1129729820928182.
73. van Rens MFPT, Hugill K, Gaffari MAK, Francia AV, Ramkumar T, Garcia KLP, et al. Outcomes of establishing a neonatal peripheral vascular access team. Arch Dis Child Fetal Neonat Ed. 2021;108(1):F88–9. https://doi.org/10.1136/fetalneonatal-2021-322764.
74. Barone G, D'Andrea V, Ancora G, Cresi F, Maggio L, Capasso A, et al. The neonatal DAV-expert algorithm: a GAVeCeLT/GAVePed consensus for the choice of the most appropriate venous access in newborns. Eur J Pediatr. 2023;182(8):3385–95. https://doi.org/10.1007/s00431-023-04984-4.
75. National Health Service, (NHS) Health Education England. Human factors and healthcare. Evidencing the impact of human factors training to support improvements in patient safety and to contribute to cultural change. 2019. https://www.hee.nhs.uk/sites/default/files/documents/Health%20Education%20England%20and%20CIEHF%20-%20Human%20Fact12   ors%20and%20Healthcare%20Report.pdf. Accessed 12 August 2024.
76. van Rens MFPT, Hugill K, Francia ALV. A new approach for early recognition of peripheral intravenous (PIV) infiltration: a pilot appraisal of a sensor technology in a neonatal population. Vasc Access. 2019;5(2):38–41. https://doi.org/10.33235/va.5.2.38-41.

77. D'Andrea V, Prontera G, Carlino R, Di Trani H, Carlettini I, Pittiruti M, et al. Optical detection of infiltration during peripheral intravenous infusion in neonates. J Vasc Access. 2023;25:1780. https://doi.org/10.1177/11297298231177723.

78. van Rens MFPT, Vijlbrief D, Braun S, Hugill K, van Loon FHJ, van de Hoogen A. Peripheral intravenous therapy infiltration/extravasation (PIVIE) risks and the potential for earlier notification of events using a novel sensor technology in a neonatal population. J Vasc Access. 2023;25:1801. https://doi.org/10.1177/11297298231185536.

79. Pittiruti M, Annetta MG, D'andrea V. Point-of-care ultrasound for vascular access in neonates and children. Eur J Pediatr. 2024;183:1073–8. https://doi.org/10.1007/s00431-023-05378-2.

80. Sobczak A, Dudzik A, Kruczek P, Kwinta P. Ultrasound monitoring of umbilical catheters in the neonatal intensive care unit—a prospective observational study. Front Pediatr. 2021;9:9. https://doi.org/10.3389/fped.2021.665214.

81. Brusciano V, Lecce M. Advantages of the use of ultrasound in newborn vascular access: a systematic review. J Ultrasound. 2024;27(2):203–7. https://doi.org/10.1007/s40477-023-00832-1.

82. Galen B, Baron S, Young S, Hall A, Berger-Spivack L, Southern W. Reducing peripherally inserted central catheters and midline catheters by training nurses in ultrasound-guided peripheral intravenous catheter placement. BMJ Qual Saf. 2020;29(3):245–9. https://doi.org/10.1136/bmjqs-2019-009923.

83. D'Andrea V, Prontera G, Rubortone SA, Pezza L, Pinna G, Barone G, et al. Umbilical venous catheter update: a narrative review including ultrasound and training. Front Pediatr. 2022;9:774705. https://doi.org/10.3389/fped.2021.774705.

84. Rubortone SA, Costa S, Perri A, D'Andrea V, Vento G, Barone G. Real-time ultrasound for tip location of umbilical venous catheter in neonates: a pre/post intervention study. Ital J Pediatr. 2021;47(1):68. https://doi.org/10.1186/s13052-021-01014-7.

85. Beam K, Sharma P, Levy P, Beam AL. Artificial intelligence in the neonatal intensive care unit: the time is now. J Perinatol. 2023; https://doi.org/10.1038/s41372-023-01718-z.

86. Helm JM, Swiergosz AM, Haeberle HS, Karnuta JM, Schaffer JL, Krebs VE, et al. Machine learning and artificial intelligence: definitions, applications, and future directions. Curr Rev Musculoskelet Med. 2020;13(1):69–76. https://doi.org/10.1007/s12178-020-09600-8.

87. McAdams RM, Kaur R, Sun Y, Bindra H, Cho SJ, Singh H. Predicting clinical outcomes using artificial intelligence and machine learning in neonatal intensive care units: a systematic review. J Perinatol. 2022;42:1561–75.

88. Saruwatari MS, Nguyen TN, Talari HF, Matisoff AJ, Sharma KV, Donoho KG, et al. Assessing the effect of augmented reality on procedural outcomes during ultrasound-guided vascular access. Ultrasound Med Biol. 2023;49(11):2346–53. https://doi.org/10.1016/j.ultrasmedbio.2023.07.011.

89. De Bie FR, Davey MG, Larson AC, Deprest J, Flake AW. Artificial placenta and womb technology: past, current, and future challenges towards clinical translation. Prenat Diagn. 2021;41(1):145–58. https://doi.org/10.1002/pd.5821.

90. Flake AW, De Bie FR, Munson DA, Feudtner C. The artificial placenta and EXTEND technologies: one of these things is not like the other. J Perinatol. 2023;43:1343–8. https://doi.org/10.1038/s41372-023-01716-2.

91. Shah NR, Mychaliska GB. The new frontier in ECLS: artificial placenta and artificial womb for premature infants. Semin Pediatr Surg. 2023;32(4):151336. https://doi.org/10.1016/j.sempedsurg.2023.151336.

92. Kukora SK, Mychaliska GB, Weiss EM. Ethical challenges in first-in-human trials of the artificial placenta and artificial womb: not all technologies are created equally, ethically. J Perinatol. 2023;43(11):1337–42. https://doi.org/10.1038/s41372-023-01713-5.

93. Romanis EC. Artificial womb technology and the frontiers of human reproduction: conceptual differences and potential implications. J Med Ethics. 2018;44(11):751–5. https://doi.org/10.1136/medethics-2018-104910.

94. Ohuma E, Moller A-B, Bradley E, Chalwere S, Hussain-Alkhateeb L, Lewin A, et al. National, regional, and worldwide estimates of preterm birth in 2020, with trends from 2010: a systematic analysis. Lancet. 2023;402(10409):1261–71. https://doi.org/10.1016/S0140-6736(23)00878-4.

95. Waddington C, van Veenendaal NR, O'Brien K, Patel N. Family integrated care: supporting parents as primary caregivers in the neonatal intensive care unit. Pediatr Investig. 2021;5(2):148–54. https://doi.org/10.1002/ped4.12277.
96. Soleimani F, Azari N, Ghiasvand H, Shahrokhi A, Rahmani N, Fatollahierad S. Do NICU developmental care improve cognitive and motor outcomes for preterm infants? A systematic review and meta-analysis. BMC Pediatr. 2020;20(1):67. https://doi.org/10.1186/s12887-020-1953-1.
97. Soni R, Tscherning C. Family-centred and developmental care on the neonatal unit. Paediatr Child Health. 2021;31(1):18–23. https://doi.org/10.1016/j.paed.2020.10.003.
98. Zanoni P, Scime NV, Benzies K, McNeil DA, Mrklas K. Facilitators and barriers to implementation of Alberta family integrated care (FICare) in level II neonatal intensive care units: a qualitative process evaluation substudy of a multicentre cluster-randomised controlled trial using the consolidated framework for implementation research. BMJ Open. 2021;11(10):e054938. https://doi.org/10.1136/bmjopen-2021-054938.
99. British Association of Perinatal Medicine (BAPM). Enhancing shared decision making in neonatal care: a BAPM framework for practice. London: BAPM; 2019.